D0266050

Consent in Surgery
A practical guide

Edited by

ROBA KHUNDKAR
Specialty Registrar, Plastic and Reconstructive Surgery
Queen Elizabeth Hospital, Birmingham

SAMANTHA DE SILVA
Specialty Registrar, Ophthalmology
John Radcliffe Hospital, Oxford

and

RAJAT CHOWDHURY
Specialty Registrar, Radiology
Southampton General Hospital, Southampton

Forewords by
JOHN BLACK
President
Royal College of Surgeons of England

and

TIM GOODACRE
Vice President
British Association of Plastic, Reconstructive and Aesthetic Surgeons

Radcliffe Publishing
Oxford • New York

Radcliffe Publishing Ltd
18 Marcham Road
Abingdon
Oxon OX14 1AA
United Kingdom

617.9
KHU

www.radcliffepublishing.com

Electronic catalogue and worldwide online ordering facility.

© 2010 Roba Khundkar, Samantha De Silva and Rajat Chowdhury
Illustrations © 2010 Daniel James

Roba Khundkar, Samantha De Silva and Rajat Chowdhury have asserted their right under the
Copyright, Designs and Patents Act 1998 to be identified as the authors of this work.

All rights reserved. No part of this publication may be reproduced, stored in a retrieval system
or transmitted, in any form or by any means, electronic, mechanical, photocopying, recording
or otherwise, without the prior permission of the copyright owner.

British Library Cataloguing in Publication Data
A catalogue record for this book is available from the British Library.

ISBN-13: 978-184619-366-8

The paper used for the text pages of this book
is FSC certified. FSC (The Forest Stewardship
Council) is an international network to promote
responsible management of the world's forests.

Mixed Sources
Product group from well-managed
forests and other controlled sources
www.fsc.org Cert no. SGS-COC-2482
© 1996 Forest Stewardship Council

FSC

Typeset by Pindar NZ, Auckland, New Zealand
Printed and bound by TJI Digital, Padstow, Cornwall, UK

Contents

Foreword

Effective communication and trust between a patient and their surgeon are essential elements of good healthcare. They are no less important to the best possible clinical outcome than the surgeon's experience and operative skills, or the care and support of nursing staff. Good communication about the various options for treatment, their main risks, likely side effects and possible complications, and the patient's expectations and concerns, is the basis of this trust. The cornerstone of this process is informed consent – the dialogue and agreement between patient and surgeon that establishes the programme for initial and ongoing care.

Much has been written in recent years about consent, not least because the public generally have become more and more knowledgeable about health and healthcare, and patients, rightly, have been increasingly able to exercise choice in the arrangements for their care. This latest book, the result of collaboration between senior trainees and consultants across the surgical specialties, and focusing on a number of common surgical procedures, is a welcome addition. It will, I hope, be helpful to all surgeons in their general approach to this issue and to those in each of the specialties with regard to specific operations.

John Black MD FRCS
President, Royal College of Surgeons of England
June 2010

Foreword

One of the abiding characteristics of late twentieth century and early new millennium society is the loss of trust in individuals, professions, and institutions. Whilst popular surveys indicate that the medical profession maintains one of the highest levels of trustworthiness by the public, most practitioners of my generation would vouch for a general erosion of trust with commensurate increasing demand for reassurance across the period of our career.

Surgical procedures must be amongst the most challenging life events that most members of society are called upon to embrace. Best surgical practice involves caring for every aspect of the management of a patient – and should extend to going even further than expected in attempting to offer the best possible experience and outcome. Part of that process includes taking care to alleviate anxiety and build trust in the surgeon and team in whom the care is vested. Good consenting procedures, whilst driven (perhaps inevitably) mostly by legal imperative to protect patients, should be seen and welcomed by surgeons as a full part of holistic care for the person seeking treatment.

This short book is a welcome guide to consent, written by authoritative voices and of digestible length. By bringing clarity to the important process, which can (unfortunately) sometimes be rushed at the beginning of a busy day, the book is of considerable value to ensuring excellence in surgical practice. Since the very best is the only standard to which all surgical teams should aspire, this volume on consent should be in every ward library, close to hand for the ever more rapidly changing teams managing surgical patients.

Tim Goodacre
Vice President, British Association of Plastic,
Reconstructive and Aesthetic Surgeons
Council Member of Medical Defence Union
June 2010

Preface

As surgeons we have a duty to provide accurate information before consent for surgery is requested. Similarly in this age of information, patients are interested in obtaining as much knowledge as possible regarding their procedure. Thus it is important that well-researched information regarding procedures is available to the surgeon in an easily available format.

Consent in Surgery explains the consent process for 52 common surgical procedures. All relevant points pertinent to the consent process for each procedure are explained, including indications, benefits, risks/complications, alternative treatment options, a brief description of the procedure and a summary of relevant scientific evidence.

The chapters describe common operations from the subspecialties of surgery including cardiothoracic surgery, neurosurgery, otolaryngology, general surgery, paediatric surgery, plastic and reconstructive surgery, trauma and orthopaedic surgery and urology.

All procedures have been specifically chosen from the Surgical Syllabus as outlined in the Intercollegiate Surgical Curriculum Project (www.iscp.ac.uk). Surgical Trainees are required to have a full understanding of these procedures to pass the MRCS exam and are also assessed on the consent procedure during interviews for higher specialist training.

We hope this book will act as a practical guide for trainees whilst consenting patients, as well as being a useful adjunct for exam and interview preparation.

Roba Khundkar
Samantha De Silva
Rajat Chowdhury
June 2010

Author's note

All figure quoted are those available from published literature. Rates may vary between surgeons, surgical techniques and hospitals. The reader is advised to familiarise him/herself with local protocols and rates if available.

Although anaesthetic risks have not been included in the complications section for each procedure, these would need to be discussed when consenting the patient. (*See* section 1.15.)

Contributors

Daniel James: illustrations
dj313@hotmail.com

Professor Gordon C Bannister
Consultant Orthopaedic Surgeon, Avon Orthopaedic Centre, Bristol

Mr Nicholas Beck
Consultant Colorectal Surgeon, Southampton General Hospital, Southampton

Professor Martin A Birchall
Professor of Laryngology, The Royal National Throat, Nose and Ear Hospital, London

Mr Marc Bullock
Specialty Registrar, General Surgery, Southampton General Hospital, Southampton

Mr Roberto P Casula
Consultant Cardiothoracic Surgeon, St Mary's Hospital, London

Miss Vivian A Elwell
Specialty Registrar, Neurosurgery, National Hospital for Neurology and Neurosurgery, London

Mr Jonathan M Fishman
Specialty Registrar, Otolaryngology, The John Radcliffe Hospital, Oxford

Dr Naaheed Mukadam
Specialty Registrar, Psychiatry, Chase Farm Hospital, London

Mr Adekoyejo Odutola
Specialty Registrar, Trauma and Orthopaedic Surgery, Bristol Royal Hospital for Children, Bristol

Mr Jeya Palan
Specialty Registrar, Trauma and Orthopaedic Surgery, Leicester Royal Infirmary, Leicester

Dr Premal Amrishkumar Patel
Specialty Registrar, Radiology, Southampton General Hospital, Southampton

Professor Agostino Pierro
Nuffield Professor of Paediatric Surgery, UCL Institute of Child Health and Great Ormond Street Hospital for Children, London

Mr Michael Phillips
Consultant Vascular Surgeon, Southampton General Hospital, Southampton

Professor John Primrose
Professor of Surgery and Honorary Consultant Surgeon, Southampton General Hospital, Southampton

Dr Anamika Sehgal
Specialty Registrar, Anaesthetics and ICM, Poole General Hospital, Poole & Royal Bournemouth Hospital, Bournemouth

Mr Joseph Thomas
Urologist, Box Hill Hospital, Melbourne

Mr Laurence D Watkins
Consultant Neurosurgeon, National Hospital for Neurology and Neurosurgery, London

Mr Paul Wilson
Consultant Plastic and Reconstructive Surgeon, Frenchay Hospital, Bristol

Introduction to consent

For treatment to be provided lawfully to a competent adult patient, he or she must consent.

1.1 Legal background

Failure to obtain consent may result in the doctor being sued for battery or negligence.

Battery: if one person touches another without consent, this may constitute battery for which damages could be awarded.

Negligence: for informed consent to be obtained a patient requires information regarding the procedure (*see* below). Failure by a doctor to give the patient certain relevant information may result in that doctor being considered negligent.

1.2 Who can obtain consent?

- The doctor providing treatment or undertaking the investigation.
- A person who is suitably trained and qualified and has sufficient knowledge of the proposed investigation or treatment, and understands the risks involved.

1.3 When is consent not required?

- If a patient is unable to consent (*see* below) and would come to harm if a procedure or intervention was not done.
- Treatment for mental illness under the Mental Health Act.
- Children (*see* below).

1.4 Valid consent: assessment of capacity

For consent to be valid, the patient must be:
  I Informed
 II Competent/have capacity
III Not be coerced

I Information

- The nature and effect of a proposed treatment must be communicated.
- Sufficient detail must be stated to enable the person consenting to understand in broad terms what is to be done.
- A doctor has a duty of care to inform a patient of risks about which any competent medical practitioner undertaking such treatment would warn a patient.
- The GMC guidelines suggest that these risks should include side effects and

complications of the potential treatment options, and failure of the intervention to achieve the stated aim.
- There is also a duty to warn of any possible serious adverse outcome, even if it is rare, and of less serious complications if they occur frequently (common practice is to inform of risks which occur in 1% or more of cases).
- A doctor is not negligent if s/he has acted in accordance with a practice accepted as proper by a responsible body of medical professionals skilled in that particular art (the 'Bolam test').

II Competence/capacity
Clinicians use the term *competence*; the legal term for this is *capacity*.
Capacity consists of the ability to:
- Understand information about the decision to be made, including what the decision is, why it needs to be made and the likely consequences of making or not making the decision.
- Retain information relevant to the decision.
- Weigh the information in order to reach a decision.
- Communicate his decision.

Communication of consent may be written or oral or by conduct (e.g. extending an arm to a doctor about to take blood, provided the doctor has explained to the patient what he wishes to do).
A patient lacking any of these abilities will lack capacity to consent to treatment.
Remember, capacity is decision-specific and time-specific. Repeated assessments of capacity may therefore be necessary if a long time has elapsed since the procedure/operation was discussed with the patient.

III Lack of coercion
Consent is not valid if it is obtained:
- By fraud, e.g. a fundamental deception regarding the nature of the act or the identity of the person who is to provide the treatment.
- By duress: consent cannot be validly obtained from a person not acting under his or her own free will.

1.5 Refusal/withdrawal
Provided the patient is competent, a refusal may be for any reason, good or bad, or for no reason at all.
A patient possessing capacity may withdraw consent at any time before the authorised treatment has been given.
If consent is withdrawn after treatment has started, the doctor must stop but cannot leave the patient in an unacceptable state.

1.6 Advance directives
A patient may express present intention to refuse treatment in specified circumstances.
Doctors are bound to comply with such statements if certain conditions are fulfilled:
- The patient must have capacity to refuse medical treatment.
- There must have been no other influence, e.g. duress, undue influence or fraud.

- The scope and effect of the refusal must have intended to cover the circumstances actually prevailing at the time when the need for treatment arises.
- The patient must be in possession of knowledge of the nature and effect of the decision being taken.

1.7 Consent in patients under 18 years old

The law is not always clear in this area.

- 16- and 17-year-olds are presumed to have capacity and therefore may consent. However, if they refuse consent, then those with parental responsibility or a court may give consent for a treatment in the patient's best interests.
- Under-16-year-olds are presumed not to have capacity.
  - Those who satisfy health professionals that they do possess capacity are termed 'Gillick competent' and may consent.
  - If a Gillick competent patient refuses consent, the situation is as for 16/17-year-olds above.
  - For children who are not Gillick competent, someone with parental responsibility (*see* below) should give consent.
  - If the parent refuses to give consent for a procedure that a doctor believes to be in the patient's best interests, the courts should be involved.
- The following people have parental responsibility as outlined in the Children Act 1989:
  - The child's parents if married to each other at the time of conception/birth.
  - The child's mother, but not the father if they were not married, unless the father has acquired parental responsibility via a Court Order or a parental responsibility agreement, or the couple subsequently marry. Recent amendment: the father of a child born on or after 1 December 2003 has parental responsibility if his name appears on the birth certificate.
  - The child's legally appointed guardian, appointed either by a court, or by a parent with parental responsibility in the event of their own death.
  - A person in whose favour a court has made a Residence Order concerning the child.
  - A Local Authority designated in a Care Order in respect of the child.
  - A Local Authority or authorised person who holds an Emergency Protection Order in respect of the child.

1.8 Consent in patients lacking capacity

Capacity refers to a person's ability to perform a specific act and not a global state. Examples of when this might be impaired include:

- cognitive impairment, e.g. dementia, delirium
- intellectual impairment
- a psychiatric condition, e.g. depression, mania
- in the event of coercion
- temporary incapacity, e.g. unconsciousness.

If possible, a doctor should try and enable patients to gain capacity to make decisions, e.g. through treatment of a psychiatric disorder.

- For adults without capacity, no other person has any power to consent or refuse

treatment on their behalf (in England), unless they have appointed a Lasting Power of Attorney.
- The doctor remains under a duty of care to provide whatever treatment is in the patient's best interests.
- In the case of temporary incapacity, the doctor must decide whether the treatment is necessary to prevent deterioration in health, or to effect an improvement in it, before the patient is likely to recover the capacity to make his own decision.

1.9 Mental Capacity Act 2005

The Mental Capacity Act (MCA) 2005 came into effect in April 2007 and provides a statutory framework for treating people who lack capacity to make decisions for themselves. It covers health and welfare decisions in England and Wales.

The MCA does not generally apply to children under the age of 16 years. Treatment of children therefore is governed by common law principles.

The MCA applies to adults and people aged 16–17 years who lack mental capacity to make decisions for themselves except that people under the age of 18 years cannot:
- make a Lasting Power of Attorney
- make an Advanced Decision to refuse treatment
- have a statutory will made for them by the Court of Protection.

If someone aged 16–17 years has capacity to make decisions for themselves but the person with parental responsibility disagrees with this decision, the Family Division of the High Court can be asked to settle the dispute.

The way the MCA affects those over the age of 18 years is summarised below:

What does the MCA cover?

COVERED BY THE MCA	NOT COVERED BY THE MCA
Everyday decisions, e.g. clothing, activities	Decisions about family relationships, e.g. marriage, sexual relations, divorce
Health-related matters	Mental Health Act-related matters
Choice of place of residence	Voting rights
General matters related to welfare	Unlawful killing/assisted suicide

The five statutory principles

These are principles that underpin the MCA, in order to protect those who lack mental capacity whilst limiting the restrictions placed upon them.
1 A person must be assumed to have capacity unless it is established that they lack capacity.
2 A person is not to be treated as unable to make a decision unless all practicable steps to help them do so have been taken without success (e.g. trying alternative forms of communication, giving more time, trying to improve capacity before final assessment).
3 A person is not to be treated as unable to make a decision merely because he makes an unwise decision.
4 An act done or decision made under the MCA, for or on behalf of a person who lacks capacity, must be done or made in their best interests.
5 Before the act is done or the decision is made, one should consider if the purpose for which it is needed can be as effectively achieved in a way that is less restrictive of the person's rights and freedom of action.

Flowcharts: capacity assessments in adults

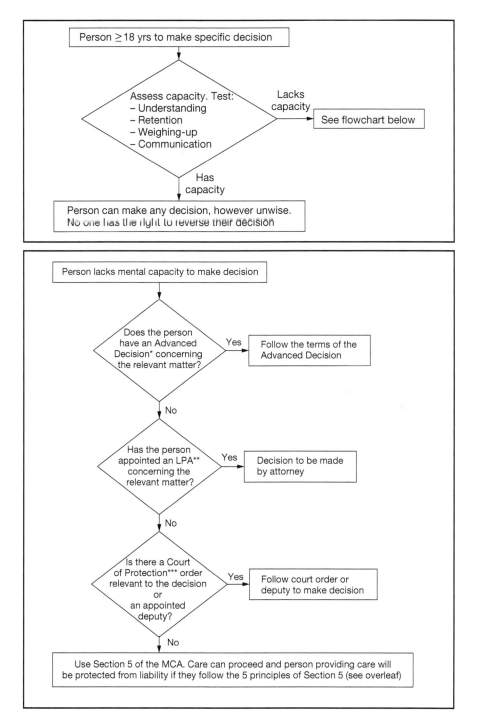

Five principles of Section 5

1 The act is one undertaken in connection with another person's care or treatment (i.e. not financial matters).
2 The person doing it takes reasonable steps to establish whether the recipient has capacity.
3 S/he reasonably believes the recipient lacks capacity relevant to the care/treatment.
4 S/he reasonably believes that it is in their *best interests* for the act to be done.
5 If s/he uses restraint, this is felt to be necessary to prevent harm to the person who lacks capacity and is proportionate to the risk and potential seriousness of that harm.

Best interests assessment

- Encourage person themselves to take part and find out their views.
- Consult others. If there are no relatives/friends involved in their care or named as someone to be consulted then you MUST consult an Independent Mental Capacity Advocate
- In an emergency situation it is usually in the person's best interests to treat without delay. The only important exception to this is when those providing treatment are satisfied there is a valid Advanced Decision in place that constitutes a refusal of treatment.

Important terms

* **Advanced Decisions (AD)** in the MCA enable people over the age of 18 years to make decisions to refuse medical treatment in the future when they may lack the capacity to make decisions about treatment. If the AD concerns life-sustaining treatment it must be
  — in writing
  — signed and witnessed, and
  — state clearly that the decision applies even if life is at risk.
** **Lasting Power of Attorney (LPA)** – a person with mental capacity to make this decision, can give another person authority to make decisions regarding financial and personal welfare matters (including healthcare) on their behalf should they lack capacity in the future. LPAs must be registered with the Public Guardian to be valid and decisions made by the attorney are as valid as ones made by the person themselves.
*** **The Court of Protection (COP)** was set up to deal with financial and welfare matters for those who lack capacity to do so themselves. Applying to the Court may be necessary in difficult cases or where disputes cannot otherwise be resolved, and fees are usually involved. The COP can decide if a person has capacity regarding a particular decision. They can make declarations, decisions or orders on matters affecting those who lack capacity or can appoint deputies to make decisions on that person's behalf. They also decide whether LPAs are valid.

Independent Mental Capacity Advocates (IMCA) are specially trained professionals appointed by the local authority (in England, and the local health board in Wales), working in partnership with NHS organisations. They support people who lack capacity in making decisions if they do not have any other support.

1.10 Mental Health Act 2007 and consent

The 2007 amendments to the Mental Health Act (MHA) 1983 came into effect in November 2008. The MHA is a legal framework for compulsory detention and treatment of people suffering with mental disorders. The person has to be:

- suffering with a mental disorder of a nature and/or degree that necessitates treatment in hospital, and this treatment is necessary
- for the person's own health and/or safety or
- for the protection of others.

The MHA cannot be used to treat people against their will for physical conditions, regardless of whether their mental disorder affects their capacity to make decisions regarding treatment. If a mental disorder is felt to affect the person's capacity, treatment for the mental disorder may need to be given in order to improve their capacity and this may need to be carried out under the MHA.

The MCA applies equally to people subject to the MHA, except:

- the MCA cannot be used to make decisions regarding treatment of the mental disorder of someone detained under the MHA
- where guardianship is in place (*see* above)
- IMCAs do not need to be involved in decisions that are made under the MHA.

1.11 Consent for audio/visual recording including photography

Specific consent should be obtained for this with clear explanations to patients if the recording is to be used for teaching, audit or research. Patients have the right to refuse consent, without their care being compromised, if this is the case.

1.12 Consent for research

Separate consent should be obtained for any research and the nature of the research should be fully explained including how it differs from the usual treatment, any risks, and available evidence for any new treatment offered.

1.13 Human Tissue Act 2004

Enforced since September 2006, this sets out the legal framework for the storage and use of tissue from the living, and removal, storage and use of tissue from the dead. The Act also established the Human Tissue Authority (HTA) responsible for approving transplantation of organs from living donors and bone marrow from adults and children who cannot consent. Appropriate informed consent is required if tissue is to be stored.

1.14 Jehovah's Witnesses

It is against the belief of Jehovah's Witnesses to receive blood products, and thus adults are able to make informed decisions to refuse these in surgical treatment. Many hospitals have a Jehovah's Witness Hospital Liaison Committee with whom these issues may be discussed. For medico-legal purposes it is advisable to obtain a signature of the patient in the notes indicating that s/he refuses blood products.

The issue of a child whose parents are Jehovah's Witnesses and refuse for the child to have blood products, is more controversial. In this instance, the courts may have to be consulted if administering blood products is in the best interest of the child.

1.15 Consenting for general anaesthesia

The overall risk of undergoing any general anaesthetic depends on patient, surgical, and anaesthetic factors. Patient factors include pre-existing cardiorespiratory or renal disease, smoking, and obesity. Surgical factors such as the length and complexity of surgery, degree of blood loss, and whether surgery is elective vs. emergency, are also important. Type of anaesthetic given to the patient, drugs used, the airway device employed, and use of regional anaesthesia, all relate to anaesthetic issues.

In general terms, the side effects and complications of a general anaesthetic can be divided into categories depending on the likelihood of occurrence. Listed below are those which may be relevant for a surgeon during consent for general anaesthesia. An anaesthetist will be able to provide more detail for individual patients.

Very common: 1 in 10 patients
- postoperative nausea and vomiting
- sore throat
- dizziness, blurred vision, feeling faint
- shivering
- headache.

Common: 1 in 100 patients
- aches, pains and backache
- confusion or memory loss.

Uncommon: 1 in 1000 patients
- chest infection or an existing medical condition getting worse
- awareness – becoming conscious during the operation
- dental damage or damage to lips, teeth and tongue.

Rare: 1 in 10 000 patients or very rare: 1 in 100 000 patients
- heart attack or cerebrovascular event (CVA)
- serious drug allergy
- death related to anaesthesia (5 per million anaesthetics in the UK).

1.16 MRSA and surgery

Methicillin resistant *Staphylococcus aureus* (MRSA) is a normal commensal organism of the human skin and nose. Up to 30% of the general population is colonised with MRSA (higher in hospital staff and patients due to contact with infected cases, and use of antibiotics). It is important to inform patients that as a carrier, they may be a source of infection themselves.

Although a colonising organism, MRSA may cause a variety of conditions including wound infections, ulcers, deep abscesses and bacteraemia. Strains of MRSA represent over 40% of all *Staphylococcus aureus* bacteraemias. The General Practice Research Database for the period 2000–04 estimated an average incidence of adult MRSA infection or colonisation of 15.2 per 100 000.

Most surgical specialties have a rate of MRSA bacteraemia between 0.5 and 1.5 cases per 10 000 patient-days, and intervention may reduce the rate of systemic and surgical site infection.

The Department of Health recommends that most elective patients are screened for MRSA on or prior to admission, and started on an appropriate decolonisation regime if found to be positive. This does not apply to children. A patient may refuse to be screened, in which case the consequence of the decision must be explained to the patient, including possible delays to their treatment.

It is worth remembering that no large clinical trial has evaluated the efficacy of such universal screening. Recent studies on screening programs to identify carriers of MRSA have been equivocal. A recent prospective randomised crossover clinical trial involving all surgical specialties (21 754 patients over a period of 18 months) within one Swiss teaching hospital examined the impact of an admission screening intervention on MRSA incidence, acquisition, and surgical site infection. In this study the MRSA admission screening strategy did not reduce nosocomial MRSA infection in a surgical department with endemic MRSA prevalence but relatively low rates of MRSA infection.

In discussing MRSA colonisation and infection with patients, it is useful to know the incidence at the hospital you work in. This should be available on the Clinical Intranet, or from the Microbiology department.

References

- Francis R, Johnston C. *Medical Treatment: decisions and the law*. London: Butterworths; 2001.
- Sidaway v. Board of Governors of the Bethlem Royal Hospital and the Maudsley Hospital [1985] AC 871 883H.
- Jameson SS, Amarasuriya UK, Vint H, *et al*. The Mental Capacity Act 2005: relevance for the surgeon. *Bull Royal Coll Surg*. 2009; **91**(5): 176–9.
- Department of Health. *Reference guide to consent for examination or treatment*. 2nd ed. London: DoH; 2009. Available at: www.dh.gov.uk/en/Publicationsandstatistics/Publications/PublicationsPolicyAndGuidance/DH_4006757 (accessed 13 June 2010).
- Wheeler R. Consent in surgery. *Ann R Coll Surg Engl*. 2006; **88**(3): 261–4.
- Office of the Public Guardian. *Mental Capacity Act (2005) Code of Practice*. London: 2007. Available at: www.publicguardian.gov.uk/mca/code-of-practice.htm (accessed 13 June 2010).
- Royal College of Anaesthetists. *Anaesthesia explained: information for patients, relatives and friends*. London: RCA; 2008. Available at: www.youranaesthetic.info (accessed 13 June 2010).
- Baker B, Jenkins K. Consent and anaesthetic risk. In: Allman KG, Wilson IH, editors. *Oxford Handbook Of Anaesthesia*. 2nd ed. Oxford: Oxford University Press; 2006. pp. 18–21.
- Department of Health. *A Simple Guide to MRSA*. London: DoH; 2007. Available at: www.dh.gov.uk/en/Publicationsandstatistics/Publications/PublicationsPolicyAndGuidance/DH_4113886 (accessed 13 June 2010).
- Schneider-Lindner V, Delaney JA, Dial S, *et al*. Antimicrobial drugs and community-acquired methicillin-resistant *Staphylococcus aureus*, United Kingdom. *Emerg Infect Dis*. 2007; **13**: 994–1000.
- Gould FK, Brindle R, Chadwick PR, *et al*. MRSA Working Party of the British Society for Antimicrobial Chemotherapy: guidelines for the prophylaxis and treatment of methicillin-resistant *Staphylococcus aureus* (MRSA) infections in the United Kingdom. *J Antimicrob Chemother*. 2009; **63**(5): 849–61.
- Meehan J, Jamali AA, Nguyen H. Prophylactic antibiotics in hip and knee arthroplasty. *J Bone Joint Surg Am*. 2009; **91**: 2480–90.
- Harbarth S, Fankhauser C, Schrenzel J, *et al*. Universal screening for methicillin-resistant *Staphylococcus aureus* at hospital admission and nosocomial infection in surgical patients. *JAMA*. 2008; **299**(10): 1149–57.

Further information

- Department of Health. *Reference Guide to Consent for Examination or Treatment*. 2nd ed. London: DoH; 2009. Available at: www.dh.gov.uk/en/Publicationsandstatistics/Publications/PublicationsPolicyAndGuidance/DH_103643 (accessed 13 June 2010).
- Church, J. *Informed Consent: a mini topic review*. Specialist Library for Surgery, Theatres and Anaesthesia, National Library for Health; April 2007. Available at: www.library.nhs.uk/Theatres/ViewResource.aspx?resID=259250 (accessed 13 June 2010).
- British Medical Association. *Consent Tool Kit*. 5th ed. London: BMA; 2009. Available at: www.bma.org.uk/images/consenttoolkitdec2009_tcm41-193139.pdf

Generic procedures

2.1 Central venous cannulation
Key points
Cannulation of large veins is most commonly carried out via an internal jugular, subclavian, or femoral approach. An antecubital fossa approach may also be used (peripherally inserted central catheter or PICC line).

Procedural considerations
- Assessment of risk factors for prolonged bleeding prior to insertion such as acquired or inherited coagulopathies, drugs such as clopidogrel, heparin and warfarin.
- Pre-procedure check of haemoglobin, platelet count and clotting function.
- Line selection
  - Use a single-lumen line unless multiple ports are needed. Consider a tunnelled or antimicrobial line.
- Method of insertion
  - Sterile procedure – gown, gloves and drape, local anaesthesia. Check line and flush all ports prior to and following insertion. Insert line using the Seldinger technique. Suture line in situ.
- Internal jugular approach
  - NICE recommends using ultrasound guidance for internal jugular vein approach.
  - The right side is often chosen because the right internal jugular vein, superior vena cava and right atrium are more directly aligned.
  - Head-down position distends the vein and reduces the risk of air embolism.
  - Patient should be in the supine position with the head turned to the contralateral side.
  - High approach (lower risk of pneumothorax): palpate the carotid artery at the level of C6/cricoid cartilage and insert a needle at 30° to the skin towards the ipsilateral nipple.
  - Once venous blood is aspirated, lower the needle in line with the vein and cannulate.

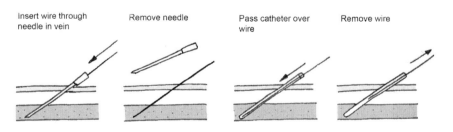

FIGURE 2.1 Central venous cannulation.

- – Low approach: insert needle at the apex of the triangle formed by the two heads of sternocleidomastoid.
- **Subclavian approach**
  - – Lowest risk of catheter-related bloodstream infections and most comfortable for the patient.
  - – Highest risk of pneumothorax or haemothorax.
  - – Contraindicated in coagulopathy as pressure cannot be easily applied to a bleeding vessel.
  - – Technique as above: insert needle 1 cm below junction of lateral two-thirds and medial one-third of the clavicle. Direct needle under the clavicle towards the suprasternal notch.
- **Femoral approach**
  - – Carries the highest risk of sepsis, but often the easier route, especially in emergencies.
  - – Technique as above: extend leg and abduct hip slightly. With finger on femoral pulse, insert needle 1–2 cm medial to artery at approximately a 45° angle.

Postoperative considerations
- Post-procedure chest X-ray if internal jugular or subclavian (or PICC) approach – the catheter tip should lie in the superior vena cava above the pericardial reflection. This is at the level of T4 or the carina on chest X-ray. Look specifically for pneumothorax or haemothorax.

Additional considerations
Line management:
- Remove line within 24 hours if not needed.
- Do not routinely change central lines.
- Remove line if infection is suspected. Send blood cultures and line tip to microbiology.
- Document daily assessment of catheter site.
- Use needle-free ports and clean site before accessing.

CONSENT FORM
Name of procedure: internal jugular/subclavian/femoral line insertion
Benefits:
> For venous access
> For administration of therapy
> For haemodialysis
> For measurement of central venous pressure and assessing volume status
> For cardiac or pulmonary vessel cannulation
> For pacemaker insertion.
Risks:
> Mechanical
> > Haematoma: 0.4%–0.6%[1]
> > Arterial puncture: 3.1%–4.9% subclavian, 6.3%–9.4% internal jugular, 9%–15% femoral[1]
> > Pneumothorax: 1.5%–3.1% subclavian approach, <0.1%–0.2% internal jugular approach[1]
> > Haemothorax: 0.4%–0.6%[1]

Infection
> May be colonisation, bloodstream infection or exit site infection.
> Risk of colonisation is low until day 5–7.[1]
> Overall incidence 2–7 episodes per 1000 catheter days.[2]
> Higher rate for femoral approach: 1.2 episodes per 1000 catheter days for subclavian vs. 4.5 episodes/1000 catheter days for femoral.[3]

Thromboembolic
> Thrombosis (1.9% subclavian, 21.5% femoral[3]) – all have potential to embolise but incidence unclear.
> Air or cannula embolus.

Arrhythmias

Procedure involves: Local anaesthesia

Key publications
McGee DC, Gould MK. Preventing complications of central venous catherization. *NEJM*. 2003; **348**: 1123–33.[1]
- A comprehensive review of complications of central venous catheterisation and potential means of minimising risks. These include:
  - Sterile barrier precautions including gown, gloves and large drape.
  - Seeking help if catheterisation is unsuccessful at the third attempt, as the incidence of mechanical complications significantly increases with further attempts.
  - Ultrasound guidance, especially for internal jugular approach.
  - If suspected arterial puncture, and not obviously identifiable by colour and pulsatility of blood, e.g. in a hypotensive patient, recommended to insert a single-lumen catheter, which does not require dilation to insert. Subsequently, samples can be sent for analysis, or catheter connected to pressure transducer to identify if arterial.
  - Close catheter hubs at all times to prevent air embolism.
  - Use of prophylactic antibiotics shown to reduce rate of infection but concern over antibiotic resistance.

References
1 McGee DC, Gould MK. Preventing complications of central venous catherization. *NEJM*. 2003; **348**: 1123–33.
2 Zingg W, Cartier-Fässler V, Walder B. Central venous catheter-associated infections. *Best Pract Res Clin Anaesthesiol*. 2008; **22**(3): 407–21.
3 Merrer J, De Jonghe B, Golliot F, *et al*. Complications of femoral and subclavian venous catheterization in critically ill patients: a randomized controlled trial. *JAMA*. 2001; **286**: 700–7.

2.2 Arterial cannulation
Key points
An arterial cannula or arterial line is most commonly inserted into the radial artery. Alternative sites include the ulnar, brachial, femoral, posterior tibial and dorsalis pedis arteries.

Anatomy – in the distal forearm the radial artery is palpated between the tendons of brachioradialis and flexor carpi radialis. The radial artery lies medial to the distal head of the radius.

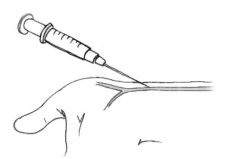

FIGURE 2.2 Arterial cannulation.

Procedural considerations
* Usually inserted in critical care setting rather than general wards as nursing staff need to be trained in line management.
* Before cannulating either the radial or ulnar artery, it is important to try and assess whether circulation to the hand will be compromised. A modified Allen's test can be performed to help assess collateral circulation. Elevate the patient's hand and compress both the radial and ulnar artery at the wrist. Ask the patient to blanch the palm by clenching and opening the hand. Release the ulnar artery if you wish to cannulate the radial artery, OR release the radial artery if you choose to cannulate the ulnar artery. The hand should re-perfuse within 5–7 seconds. Over 15 seconds is considered abnormal and an alternative site for cannulation may need to be considered. Although this test is used widely it has a poor predictive value.
* Check all equipment is ready for attachment to cannula once inserted.
* Supinate the forearm, and hyperextend the wrist.
* Sterile technique.
* Palpate the radial artery.
* Local anaesthesia (may not be required if patient has impaired consciousness or is sedated, for example, in an intensive care environment).
* An arterial cannula can be sited using the Seldinger technique. Insert the introducer needle into the radial artery at an angle of 45° until a flashback is seen. Advance the guide-wire through the introducer needle and holding onto the distal end of the guide-wire, remove the introducer needle. Pass the arterial cannula over the guide-wire so it is located within the radial artery. Finally, remove the guide-wire.
* An arterial cannula can also be sited using a similar technique to that used for peripheral venous access.

Postoperative considerations
* Check for blood flow and flush with saline (can contain heparin).
* Apply a small sterile dressing and secure well.
* Clearly label the cannula and line as ARTERIAL to distinguish it from venous access.
* Ensure the transducer is zeroed and at the level of the patient's heart. Check for an appropriate arterial trace.

Additional considerations
Contraindications:
* Inadequate peripheral circulation.
* Buerger's disease/Raynaud's disease.

- Burn or infection over site of access.
- Relative contraindications: uncontrolled coagulopathy.

CONSENT FORM
Name of procedure: Arterial cannulation/arterial line insertion
Benefits:
    Arterial blood gas sampling
    Invasive blood pressure monitoring
    Cardiac output monitoring
    Frequent blood sampling
Risks:[1]
    Artery occlusion (temporary)
        radial: range 1.5%–35%, mean 19.2%
        femoral: 1.45%
    Permanent ischaemia
        radial: 0.09%
        femoral: 0.18%
    Haematoma
        radial: 14.4%
        femoral: 6.1%
    Bleeding
        radial: 0.53%
        femoral: 1.58%
    Localised infection
        radial: 0.72%
        femoral: 0.78%
    Sepsis
        radial: 0.13%
        femoral: 0.44%
    Pseudoaneurysm formation
        radial: 0.09%
        femoral: 0.3%
    Rare[2]
        median nerve paralysis
        air embolism
        compartment syndrome
        carpal tunnel syndrome
Procedure involves: Local anaesthesia

Key publications
Scheer B, Perel A, Pfeiffer UJ. Clinical review: complications and risk factors of peripheral arterial catheters used for haemodynamic monitoring in anaesthesia and intensive care medicine. *Crit Care.* 2002; **6**(3): 199–204.[1]
- An extensive review of published literature from 1978 to 2001 of radial, femoral and axillary artery cannulation, including a total of 19 617 procedures.
- Complication rates are as quoted above.
- The main complication rate is of temporary radial artery occlusion, however permanent ischaemic damage as a result was much more infrequent.

References

1 Scheer B, Perel A, Pfeiffer UJ. Clinical review: complications and risk factors of peripheral arterial catheters used for haemodynamic monitoring in anaesthesia and intensive care medicine. *Crit Care*. 2002; **6**(3): 199–204.

2 Sawyer TL, Ridout R. Radial artery cannulation. Available at: http://emedicine. medscape.com/article/80450-overview (accessed 13 June 2010).

2.3 Insertion of chest drain

Key points

A chest drain or tube thoracostomy is a conduit inserted into the pleural space to remove fluid or air.

Indications include:

- Pneumothorax – following needle aspiration for a tension pneumothorax and recurrent pneumothoraces.
- Traumatic haemo/pneumothorax.
- Drainage of pleural effusion or empyema.
- Postoperatively, for example, following cardiothoracic surgery.

Procedural considerations

- Assessment of bleeding risk such as acquired or inherited coagulopathies, or anticoagulant medication such as heparin and warfarin.
- Consider ultrasound for pleural effusions – to mark a point where drain should be inserted.
- Position: lying on the bed with the ipsilateral arm behind the patient's head to expose the axilla OR sitting upright leaning over a table with a pillow.
- Site of insertion usually between 4th to 7th intercostal space, between anterior axillary and mid-axillary line.
- Aseptic technique.
- Local anaesthesia infiltration down to periosteum of chosen rib.
- Needle is advanced above the rib to avoid the neurovascular bundle.
- Before inserting the needle in a ventilated patient, allow a pause to reduce the risk of a pneumothorax.
- Use Seldinger technique to insert small bore drains. Advance a needle attached to a syringe until air or fluid is aspirated. Disconnect the syringe and feed the guide-wire

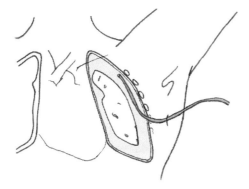

FIGURE 2.3 Insertion of chest drain.

through the needle. Pass catheter over guide-wire and remove. Insert drain into the pleural cavity and direct towards the apex.
- Suture to secure drain and apply a dressing.
- Connect to drainage system, most commonly an underwater seal device. This should be kept below level of insertion of drain. Respiratory swing of fluid in chest drain helps to confirm patency and position.

Postoperative considerations
- Chest X-ray to check position and effect of drain insertion.
- Drain can be removed 24 hours after cessation of fluid or air loss.
- Repeat chest X-ray after drain removal.

Additional considerations
- Large bore drains are useful for large fluid collections and pneumothoraces. Incise skin and use blunt dissection with artery forceps to pleura. Using a finger, sweep the area to ensure no adherent lung in the area. Insert chest drain, remove trocar and then advance drain.
- For patients at high risk of trauma due to drain insertion consider ultrasound-guided or CT-guided drain insertion.

CONSENT FORM
Name of procedure: Insertion of left/right sided chest drain
Benefits:
  Drain air/blood/fluid/pus from pleural space
Risks:
  Insertional:
    Pain 5%[3] (Seldinger technique) – 50%[4] (large bore)
    Pneumothorax: 4%[2,3]
    Bleeding: 1%[3]
    Surgical emphysema: 6%[2]
    Aberrant placement leading to visceral damage (large bore): 0.2%–6%[3]
    (Vagally mediated bradycardia)
  Infective:
    Empyema: 2%[2]
  Late:
    Dislodged drains: 6% (after 2.3 days)[2] – 21%[3]
    Blocked drains: 9%[3] – 15%[2]
    (Post-expansion pulmonary oedema)
Procedure involves: Local anaesthesia

Key publications
Davies HE, Merchant S, McGown A. A study of the complications of small bore 'Seldinger' intercostal chest drains. *Respirology.* 2008; **13**(4): 603–7. Epub 2008 Apr 14.[3]
- Most of the literature on complications of chest drains relates to large bore drains; this is a retrospective review of 100 chest drains inserted using the Seldinger technique.
- The main complications were displacement of drains (21%) and blockage of drains (9%), the latter being reduced with frequent flushing of the drain.

References

1 Laws D, Neville E, Duffy J. BTS guidelines for the insertion of a chest drain. *Thorax.* 2003; **58**(Suppl. 2): ii53–ii9.
2 Horsley A, Jones L, White J, Henry M. Efficacy and complications of small-bore, wire-guided chest drains. *Chest.* 2006; **130**(6): 1857–63.
3 Davies HE, Merchant S, McGown A. A study of the complications of small bore 'Seldinger' intercostal chest drains. *Respirology.* 2008; **13**(4): 603–7. Epub 2008 Apr 14.
3 Luketich JD, Kiss MD, Hershey J, *et al.* Chest tube insertion: a prospective evaluation of pain management. *Clin J Pain.* 1998; **14**: 152–4.

3

Cardiac surgery

3.1 Coronary artery bypass grafting

Key points

Coronary artery bypass grafting (CABG) is an operation performed to bypass athero-sclerotic narrowing in coronary arteries and improve the circulation to the myocardium.

Indications include disease of the left main coronary artery, disease of all three coron-ary vessels with or without left ventricular impairment, diffuse disease not amenable to treatment with percutaneous coronary intervention, and other high-risk patients with severe ventricular dysfunction or diabetes mellitus.[1]

The commonest grafts include saphenous vein, radial artery, and internal mammary artery (IMA). Single, double, triple, quadruple, or quintuple bypasses may be performed in the same procedure. Successful grafts to the left anterior descending coronary artery (LAD) typically last between 10 and 15 years. Any other combination of graft to non-LAD targets has shown a shorter patency rate.

Procedural considerations

- General anaesthesia and midline sternotomy.
- The procedure may be carried out 'on-pump', i.e. the heart is stopped during the operation and circulation is maintained by a cardiopulmonary bypass pump. The

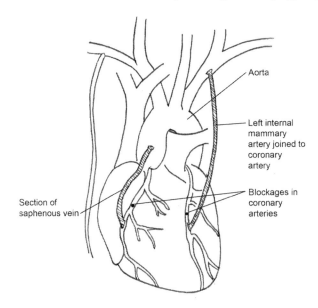

FIGURE 3.1 Coronary artery bypass graft.

18

alternative is 'off-pump' (OPCAB) in which the heart continues to beat throughout the operation.
- Saphenous vein harvesting: great saphenous vein removed from leg and used for graft/conduit. Scar down medial aspect of leg.
- Radial artery harvesting: radial artery used from non-dominant arm if collateral ulnar artery circulation is adequate (Allen's test). Contraindications include Raynaud's disease and haemodialysis patients with an arteriovenous fistula. Scar down medial aspect of forearm.
- IMA: typically used to bypass the left anterior descending (LAD) artery.
- Sternotomy is closed with wires, dissolvable skin sutures, and typically with 2–3 drains.
- Cardiac pacing wires are sited during the operation, and are removed postoperatively.
- Drains may be sited at the graft harvest wound sites.

Postoperative considerations
- Cardiac ICU for the first day followed by HDU.
- Cardiac drug infusions including nitrates for the first day with subsequent conversion to oral beta-blockers to continue for 6–12 months.
- Urinary catheterisation.
- Regular dressing changes of sternotomy and graft harvest wound sites until discharge.
- Removal of drains as output reduces, typically 24–48 hours post surgery.
- Typical hospital stay is 5–7 days.

Additional considerations
- Minimally invasive direct coronary artery bypass (MIDCAB) – performed through a smaller incision usually with the heart beating and off-pump. It is primarily indicated for LAD and right coronary artery lesions with the IMA as the graft of choice. This technique causes fewer complications, less pain after surgery, and faster recovery. Hospital stay is usually 3–4 days.

CONSENT FORM

Name of procedure: Coronary artery bypass with saphenous vein/radial artery/ internal mammary artery graft

Indications:
  Improve coronary circulation and reduce risk of myocardial infarction and death
  Relieve symptoms (angina and/or shortness of breath)

Risks:
  General:
  Bleeding: (5% reoperation for bleeding)[2]
  Infection
  Stroke: 1%–2%[2]
  Myocardial infarction: 5%–15%[2]
  Acute renal failure: 5%[2]
  DVT/PE: 0.5%[2]
  Death: 3%[2]

Specific:
> Post-perfusion syndrome (transient neurocognitive impairment associated with cardiopulmonary bypass)
> Non-union of sternum
> Keloid scarring (especially in chest)
> Chest pain recurrence
> Late graft stenosis

Procedure involves:
> General anaesthesia
> +/– cardiopulmonary bypass pump
> +/– blood transfusion

Key publications

Toumpoulis IK, Anagnostopoulos CE, Swistel DG, *et al*. Does EuroSCORE predict length of stay and specific postoperative complications after cardiac surgery? *Eur J Cardiothorac Surg*. 2005; **27**(1): 128–33.[3]
* Prospective study: 5051 CABG patients were assessed with the EuroSCORE cardiac surgery risk model and the EuroSCORE was shown to have very good discriminatory ability and calibration in predicting in-hospital mortality, sepsis and/ or endocarditis, 3-month mortality, prolonged length of stay, and respiratory failure. It was found however to be unable to predict complications including intraoperative stroke, stroke over 24 hours, postoperative myocardial infarction, deep sternal wound infection, gastrointestinal complications and re-exploration for bleeding.

SoS Investigators. Coronary artery bypass surgery vs. percutaneous coronary intervention with stent implantation in patients with multivessel coronary artery disease (the Stent or Surgery trial): a randomised controlled trial. *Lancet*. 2002; **360**(9338): 965–70.
* RCT: symptomatic patients with multivessel coronary disease – 500 patients randomised to CABG and 488 randomised to stent-assisted PCI across 53 centres in Europe and Canada.
* Primary outcome – rates of repeat revascularisation; secondary outcomes – death, Q-wave MI, all cause mortality.
* Minimum follow-up 1 year, median follow-up 2 years.
* Results: 21% of patients in the PCI group required additional revascularisation procedures compared with 6% in CABG group. The incidence of death or Q-wave myocardial infarction was similar in both groups.

Serruys PW, Morice MC, Kappetein AP, *et al*. Percutaneous coronary intervention vs. coronary-artery bypass grafting for severe coronary artery disease. *N Engl J Med*. 2009; **360**(10): 961–72.
* RCT SYNTAX trial: 1800 patients with multivessel coronary disease comparing CABG vs. PCI using drug-eluting stents (DES).
* Findings: rates of major adverse cardiac or cerebrovascular events at 12 months were significantly higher in the DES group (17.8% vs. 12.4% for CABG).

References

1 Eagle KA, Guyton RA, Davidoff R, *et al*. (Committee to update the 1999 guidelines for coronary artery bypass graft surgery). ACC/AHA 2004 guideline update for coronary

artery bypass graft surgery: a report of the American College of Cardiology/American Heart Association Task Force on Practice Guidelines. *Circulation*. 2004; **110**(14): e340–437.

2 Hogue C, Sundt T, Barzilai B, *et al*. Cardiac and neurologic complications identify risks for mortality for both men and women undergoing coronary artery bypass graft surgery. *Anesthesiology*. 2001; **95**(5): 1074–8.

3 Toumpoulis IK, Anagnostopoulos CE, Swistel DG, *et al*. Does EuroSCORE predict length of stay and specific postoperative complications after cardiac surgery? *Eur J Cardiothorac Surg*. 2005; **27**(1): 128–33.

3.2 Heart valve replacement: aortic and mitral

Key points

Heart valve replacement surgery is performed to treat valvular heart disease,[1] most commonly damaged aortic and mitral valves.

Replacement valves may be biological or mechanical prostheses. Biological valves last for approximately 10 years. Their durability is longer the older the patient, and in the more superior aortic position compared with the more inferior mitral position. Mechanical valves require lifelong anticoagulation and can last for a lifetime but are exposed to a risk of prosthetic valve endocarditis and thrombosis.

Procedural considerations

- General anaesthesia and most commonly midline sternotomy.
- 'On-pump' – the heart is stopped during the operation and circulation is maintained by a cardiopulmonary bypass pump.
- Diseased valve is excised and replacement valve is sutured into place.
- Perfusion of the heart is restarted and normal circulation restored.
- Sternotomy is closed with wires, dissolvable skin sutures, chest drains and temporary pacing wires.

Postoperative considerations

- Cardiac ICU for the first 24 hours followed by HDU.
- Anticoagulation (lifelong for mechanical valves and 3 months for biological valves and repairs).
- Urinary catheterisation.
- Physiotherapy.
- Regular dressing changes of sternotomy wound site until healed.
- Typical hospital stay is 7 days.

Additional considerations

- Keyhole surgery – performed through a smaller incision.[2]
- Percutaneous valve replacement – accessed via femoral vessels.[3]
- Alternative procedures – repair of valve and widening of a narrowed valve.

CONSENT FORM

Name of procedure: Heart valve replacement: biological or mechanical prosthesis

Benefits:
> Treat heart valve disease
> Relieve symptoms
> Increased life expectancy

Risks:

> **General:**
>> Bleeding: 12% biological AVR, 41% mechanical AVR[4]
>> Infections, chest infections
>> Stroke: 4% AVR, up to 1%/year with mechanical MVR[4]
>> Myocardial infarction (rare)
>> Acute renal failure
>> DVT/PE (rare)
>> Death
>> Risks of general anaesthesia

> **Specific:**
>> Dysrhythmia (atrial fibrillation)
>> Re-exploration: 25% biological AVR, 3% mechanical AVR[4]
>> Paravalvular leak
>> Post-perfusion syndrome (transient neurocognitive impairment associated with cardiopulmonary bypass)
>> Sternal dehiscence/infection
>> Keloid scarring (especially in chest)

Procedure involves:
> General anaesthesia
> +/– cardiopulmonary bypass pump (all cases apart from Transcatheter Aortic Valve Implantation)
> +/– blood transfusion

Key publications

Aortic valve replacement

Tabata M, Umakanthan R, Cohn LH, *et al*. Early and late outcomes of 1000 minimally invasive aortic valve operations. *Eur J Cardiothorac Surg*. 2008; **33**(4): 537–41.[5]

- Retrospective study.
- 1005 patients (median age 68) underwent minimally invasive aortic valve surgery.
- Operative mortality was 1.9%.
- Deep sternal wound infection 0.5%.
- Pneumonia 1.3%.
- Reoperation for bleeding 2.4%.
- Median length of stay was 6 days and 72% were discharged home.
- Actuarial survival was 91% at 5 years and 88% at 10 years.

van Geldorp MW, Eric Jamieson WR, Kappetein AP, *et al*. Patient outcome after aortic valve replacement with a mechanical or biological prosthesis: weighing lifetime anticoagulant-related event risk against reoperation risk. *J Thorac Cardiovasc Surg*. 2009; **137**(4): 881–6.[6]

- Retrospective study.

- 3934 patients underwent AVR with either a biological or a mechanical prosthesis between 1982 and 2003.
- Follow-up: 6.1 years in the biological arm and 8.5 years in the mechanical arm.
- Biological vs. mechanical AVR:
  - life expectancy was 11.9 years vs. 12.2 years
  - event-free life expectancy was 9.8 years vs. 9.3 years
  - reoperation-free life expectancy was 10.5 years vs. 11.9 years
  - lifetime risk of reoperation was 25% vs. 3%
  - lifetime risk of bleeding was 12% vs. 41%.

Mitral valve replacement

Kulik A, Bédard P, Lam BK, *et al*. Mechanical versus bioprosthetic valve replacement in middle-aged patients. *Eur J Cardiothorac Surg*. 2006; **30**(3): 485–91.[7]

Cohort study of long-term outcomes of mechanical vs. bioprosthetic valves in middle-aged patients.

- 659 patients aged 50–65 years who had first-time AVR and/or MVR.
- 10-year survival was 73.2 +/– 4.2% after mechanical AVR, 75.1 +/– 12.6% after bioprosthetic AVR, 74.1 +/– 4.6% after mechanical MVR, 77.9 +/– 7.4% after bioprosthetic MVR.
- 10-year reoperation rates were 35.4% and 21.3% with aortic and mitral bioprostheses, respectively.
- Major bleeding and thromboembolic events were more common following mechanical MVR.

References

1 Bonow RO, Carabello BA, Kanu C, *et al*. ACC/AHA 2006 guidelines for the management of patients with valvular heart disease: a report of the American College of Cardiology/American Heart Association Task Force on Practice Guidelines. *Circulation*. 2006; **114**(5): e84–231.
2 Deeba S, Aggarwal R, Sains P, *et al*. Cardiac robotics: a review and St. Mary's experience. *Int J Med Robot*. 2006; **2**(1): 16–20.
3 Wong MC, Clark DJ, Horrigan MC, *et al*. Advances in percutaneous treatment for adult valvular heart disease. *Intern Med J*. 2009; **39**(7): 465–74.
4 Yuh DD, Vricella LA, Baumgartner W, editors. *The Johns Hopkins Manual of Cardiothoracic Surgery*. Baltimore, MD: McGraw-Hill; 2007.
5 Tabata M, Umakanthan R, Cohn LH, *et al*. Early and late outcomes of 1000 minimally invasive aortic valve operations. *Eur J Cardiothorac Surg*. 2008; **33**(4): 537–41.
6 van Geldorp MW, Eric Jamieson WR, Kappetein AP, *et al*. Patient outcome after aortic valve replacement with a mechanical or biological prosthesis: weighing lifetime anticoagulant-related event risk against reoperation risk. *J Thorac Cardiovasc Surg*. 2009; **137**(4): 881–6.
7 Kulik A, Bédard P, Lam BK, *et al*. Mechanical versus bioprosthetic valve replacement in middle-aged patients. *Eur J Cardiothorac Surg*. 2006; **30**(3): 485–91.

General surgery

4.1 Appendicectomy: open and laparoscopic
Key points
Appendicectomy is the surgical excision of the vermiform appendix. Appendicitis is the commonest indication for emergency abdominal surgery in the UK.

The operation may be performed as an open or laparoscopic procedure. The cosmetic result is superior with laparoscopic surgery, which is the preferred method if the diagnosis is uncertain. However, the open approach may be more suitable if complicated appendicitis is anticipated or if a pneumoperitonum will be tolerated poorly due to cardiorespiratory compromise.

Procedural considerations
- General anaesthesia with induction antibiotics.
- Open techniques
  - McBurney's point lies one-third of the way along an imaginary line between the right anterior superior iliac spine and the umbilicus. McBurney's incision is 3–5 cm long at McBurney's point running perpendicular to the imaginary line described above.
  - The Lanz incision produces a better cosmetic result but is less easy to extend should the need arise.
  - The layers of the anterior abdominal wall are divided to reveal the peritoneum, which is carefully opened. The caecum is delivered into the wound along with the appendix. The appendiceal artery is ligated, the appendix base divided and the stump buried before the caecum is returned to the abdomen. The wound is closed in layers with absorbable sutures. A drain may be required for complicated appendicitis (faecal or purulent contamination).
- **Laparoscopic technique**
  - Traditionally, a 10 mm infra-umbilical port is used for laparoscope access and to create the pneumoperitoneum. A minimum of two further 5 mm ports are then

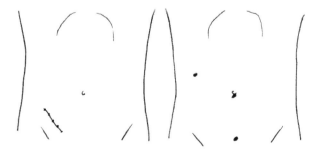

FIGURE 4.1 Incisions for appendicectomy.

inserted under direct vision. Numerous triangular configurations are possible, with the ports and the appendix lying at the vertices.

Postoperative considerations
- Free fluids orally and full diet the next day.
- DVT prophylaxis.

Additional considerations
- Pregnancy and appendicitis: appendicitis occurs in between 0.015% and 0.21% of pregnancies. Foetal mortality ranges from 0%–1.5% in simple appendicitis to 20%–35% if the appendix is perforated.[1]
- In children there appears to be no significant difference between open and laparoscopic appendicectomy regarding incidence of postoperative intra-abdominal sepsis and pain, although the open approach is more frequently associated with wound infection.[4]
- A delayed presentation may result in the presence of an appendix mass. If the patient is otherwise well, the initial management is conservative followed by an interval appendicectomy once the inflammatory process has subsided.

CONSENT FORM
Name of procedure: Appendicectomy (open or laparoscopic)
Benefits:
> Treatment of acute appendicitis
> Relieve symptoms
> Prevent disease progression including abscess formation, perforation and peritonitis.

Risks:
> Infection of surgical wound: open 7.3%, laparoscopic 3.6%[4]
> Intra-abdominal abscess: open 0.6%, laparoscopic 1.6%[4]
> Gastrointestinal complications – including ileus/small bowel obstruction/nausea and vomiting: open 4.5%, laparoscopic 3.6%[2]
> Intraoperative complications – including visceral injury and bleeding: open 0.4%, laparoscopic 0.3%[2]
> Conversion of laparoscopic to open: 5%–25% depending on the presence of complicated/perforated appendicitis[3]

Procedure involves: General anaesthesia and antibiotics

Key publications
Sauerland S, Lefering R, Neugebauer EAM. Laparoscopic versus open surgery for suspected appendicitis. Cochrane Database Syst Rev. 2004; 4: CD001546.[4]
- A systematic review of 54 RCTs comparing the therapeutic and diagnostic effects of open appendicectomy and laparoscopic appendicectomy.
- The laparoscopic approach results in less postoperative pain, fewer wound complications (OR 0.45), a shorter hospital stay and quicker return to normal activity. However, the data also suggests that there may be an increased risk of intra-abdominal sepsis associated with laparoscopic surgery (OR 2.45). The laparoscopic approach also reduces the frequency of negative appendicectomy.

Andersen BR, Kallehave FL, Andersen HK. Antibiotics versus placebo for prevention of postoperative infection after appendicectomy. Cochrane Database Syst Rev. 2005; 3: CD001439.[5]

- A systematic review of 45 RCTs and controlled clinical trials comparing any antibiotic regime with a placebo, in patients suspected of having appendicitis and who subsequently undergo appendicectomy.
- Antibiotics effectively reduce postoperative complications in patients who have undergone appendicectomy, regardless of whether they are administered pre-, peri- or postoperatively.
- The review did not compare the efficacy of single- and multidose strategies nor did it compare different antimicrobial agents. The optimum duration of antibiotics following negative, simple and complicated appendicectomy is not clear.

References

1 Guttman R, Goldman RD, Koren G. Appendicitis during pregnancy. *Can Fam Physician*. 2004; **50**: 355–7.
2 Guller U, Hervey S, Purves H, *et al*. Laparoscopic vs. open appendicectomy: outcomes comparison based on a large administrative database. *Ann Surg*. 2004; **239**: 43–52.
3 Prystowsky JB, Pugh CM, Nagle AP. Appendicitis. *Curr Probl Surg*. 2005; **42**: 694–742.
4 Sauerland S, Lefering R, Neugebauer EAM. Laparoscopic versus open surgery for suspected appendicitis. Cochrane Database Syst Rev. 2004; 4: CD001546.
5 Andersen BR, Kallehave FL, Andersen HK. Antibiotics versus placebo for prevention of postoperative infection after appendicectomy. Cochrane Database Syst Rev. 2005; 3: CD001439.

4.2 Cholecystectomy: open and laparoscopic
Key points

Cholecystectomy is the surgical excision of the gallbladder. In the UK approximately 50 000 procedures are performed each year, the majority of which are laparoscopic. The main indication for cholecystectomy is the presence of symptomatic gallstones (ranging from biliary colic to gallstone pancreatitis).

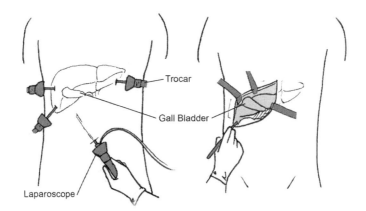

FIGURE 4.2 Cholecystectomy.

Procedural considerations

- General anaesthesia.
- Performed either during the index admission for acute cholecystitis or gallstone pancreatitis, or electively as a day-case procedure.
- Laparoscopic technique
  - Usually four 5–10 mm ports are used (umbilicus, epigastrium, right midclavicular line, right anterior axillary line). The fundus of the gallbladder is gently retracted up and over the liver. Careful dissection of Calot's triangle is essential in order to identify the cystic artery and to clarify the position of the cystic duct. Once these structures have been clipped, the gallbladder can be dissected free from the liver and delivered from the abdomen. The wound is closed with absorbable sutures. Current developments include the single incision and natural orifice surgery.
- Open techniques
  - Kocher's incision (10–18 cm right subcostal incision). The wound closed in layers with absorbable sutures.

Postoperative considerations

- Day case: day-case surgery is safe and effective for those with minimal co-morbidity and living in close proximity to the hospital, as the serious complications of cholecystectomy are either apparent at the time of surgery or do not become apparent for several days.[1]

Additional considerations

Evidence of common bile duct stones should be sought preoperatively from the clinical history, liver function tests and ultrasound. If suspicious MRCP imaging of the biliary tree may suggest the need for preoperative ERCP. Laparoscopic cholecystectomy may be accompanied by routine or selective on-table cholangiography. If common bile duct stones are identified at this stage, bile duct exploration or postoperative ERCP may be indicated although smaller stones (<5 mm) will normally pass.

CONSENT FORM

Name of procedure: Laparoscopic cholecystectomy

Benefits:
  Treatment of symptomatic gallstones

Risks:
  General:
    Wound infection – rare in the absence of drains
  Specific:
    Bile leak: 1%[3]
    Common bile duct injury: 0.2%–0.8%[4]
    Visceral injury: 0.2%[4]
    Major vessel injury: 0.07%–0.4%[4]
    Gallstone spillage: 10%–30% (of which 1.4%–5% have symptoms)[4]
    Biliary stricture – rare
    Conversion to open surgery: 2%–10%[5]

Procedure involves: General anaesthesia

- The routine use of postoperative drains is controversial. It has been argued that drain placement may help to identify bile duct injuries and prevent intra-abdominal collections. However meta-analysis demonstrates that the use of drains is associated with a prolonged hospital stay and an increased risk of wound infection without identifying any specific benefits.[2]

Key publications
- Gurusamy KS, Samraj K. Early versus delayed laparoscopic cholecystectomy for acute cholecystitis. Cochrane Database Syst Rev. 2006; 4: CD005440.[6]
  - A systematic review of five randomised trials comparing the outcome of early surgery for cholecystitis (within 7 days of the onset of symptoms) with delayed surgery (more than 6 weeks after the index admission).
  - It has become commonplace for laparoscopic cholecystectomy to be performed in the presence of active gallbladder inflammation, as contrary to traditional practice, this study demonstrates that early surgery does not significantly increase morbidity or lead to more frequent conversion to open surgery. In addition overall hospital stay may be reduced by performing surgery during the index admission.
  - Furthermore, the study emphasises the avoidable risk of gallstone-related symptoms during the interval to surgery. In the five studies under scrutiny here, 17.5% of patients in the delayed surgery group required emergency surgery because of non-resolution or recurrent cholecystitis. Conversion to open surgery is frequently necessary in this context.

References
1 Gurusamy KS, Junnarkar S, Farouk M, *et al*. Day-case versus overnight stay for laparoscopic cholecystectomy. Cochrane Database Syst Rev. 2008; 3: CD006798.
2 Gurusamy KS, Samraj K, Mullerat P, *et al*. Routine abdominal drainage for uncomplicated laparoscopic cholecystectomy. Cochrane Database Syst Rev. 2007; 4: CD006004.
3 Barkun AN, Rezieg M, Mehta SN, *et al*. McGill Gallstone Treatment Group. Postcholecystectomy biliary leaks in the laparoscopic era: risk factors, presentation, and management. *Gastrointest Endosc*. 1997; **45**: 277–82.
4 Shamiyeh A, Wayand W. Laparoscopic cholecystectomy: early and late complications and their treatment. *Langenbecks Arch Surg*. 2004; **389**: 164–71.
5 Karanjia N, Ali T. Gallstones. *Surgery*. 2007; **25**: 16–21.
6 Gurusamy KS, Samraj K. Early versus delayed laparoscopic cholecystectomy for acute cholecystitis. Cochrane Database Syst Rev. 2006; 4: CD005440.

4.3 Hartmann's procedure and sigmoid colectomy
Key points
Hartmann's procedure involves the excision of the upper two-thirds of the rectum and sigmoid colon and the formation of an end colostomy in the left iliac fossa leaving the oversewn lower third of the rectum in situ. It is the gold standard operation for complicated diverticular disease. It is also used to treat other conditions affecting the sigmoid colon and upper rectum including neoplasia, iatrogenic perforation, trauma, strictures, volvulus and anastomotic breakdown. The advantage of Hartmann's procedure is that inflammation is permitted to settle after the removal of the diseased segment of bowel, thereby optimising conditions for the restoration of gastrointestinal continuity at a later date.

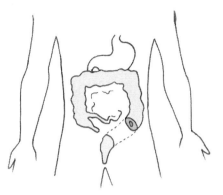

FIGURE 4.3 Hartmann's procedure.

Procedural considerations
- Preoperative resuscitation in the emergency setting is essential.
- Preoperative tests: FBC, electrolytes, clotting, renal function, group and save, ECG. Respiratory function and Echo will depend on the patient's co-morbidity and the urgency of surgery.
- General anaesthesia.
- Lower midline laparotomy incision.
- In the presence of purulent or faecal contamination, generous irrigation of the abdominal cavity is essential.

Postoperative considerations
- ITU/HDU/ward.
- Intravenous antibiotics – particularly in the presence of faecal or purulent contamination.
- Stoma training.
- Timing/appropriateness of stoma reversal.

Additional considerations
Alternative treatments:
- Colonic resection with primary anastomosis (RPA): primary restoration of gastrointestinal continuity is a viable alternative to Hartmann's procedure in certain cases. RPA is more likely to be performed in the elective setting and by dedicated colorectal surgeons, whereas Hartmann's is more frequently performed in the emergency context and particularly in the presence of significant co-morbidity or heavy intra-abdominal contamination.[1] In addition, there is considerable morbidity associated with stoma reversal which should be considered at the time of the index procedure.[2]
- Laparoscopic washout for complicated diverticulitis except in the presence of faecal contamination. Mortality and morbidity has been shown to compare favourably with open surgery, but experience is limited.[3]

CONSENT FORM

Name of procedure: Hartmann's procedure

Benefits:

> Treatment of life-threatening sepsis, colonic obstruction or enteric fistulation caused by rectal or sigmoid diverticular disease or neoplasia

Risks:

General:

> DVT/PE: 1.8%[1]
>
> MI: 5%[1]
>
> Pneumonia: 27.5%[1]
>
> CVA: 1.8%[1]
>
> Death – the overall in-hospital mortality rate for Hartmann's procedure is 20.1% rising to 23.9% for emergency procedures.[4]

Specific:

> Minor – complications not requiring surgical intervention:[1]
>
> > Wound infection: 21%
> >
> > Ileus: 0.6%
> >
> > Haemorrhage: 3%
> >
> > Stoma-related complications including retraction, necrosis, leakage, herniation, stenosis and abscess formation: 6.6%
>
> Major – complications requiring surgical intervention:
>
> > Sepsis or severe wound infection: 8.4%
> >
> > Intraperitoneal leak from stump or stoma: 3%
> >
> > Intra-abdominal haemorrhage: 3%
> >
> > Bowel obstruction: 0.6%

Procedure involves: General/regional/local anaesthesia

Key publications

David GG, Al-Sarira AA, Willmott S, *et al*. Use of Hartmann's procedure in England. *Colorectal Dis*. 2008; **11**: 308–12.[4]

- A retrospective cohort analysis of the use of Hartmann's procedure in English hospitals between April 2001 and March 2002. Data drawn from Department of health statistics.
- 3950 procedures were performed of which 72% were performed in the emergency setting.
- 72.5% of emergency Hartmann's procedures were performed for complicated diverticular disease.
- 23.3% of patients underwent reversal of Hartmann's in the subsequent 4 years of follow-up.

Constantinides VA, Tekkis PP, Senapati A. Prospective multicentre evaluation of adverse outcomes following treatment for complicated diverticular disease. *Br J Surg*. 2006; **93**: 1503–13.[1]

- A prospective multicentre trial conducted over a twelve-month period comparing adverse events from RPA surgery and Hartmann's procedure; prepared on behalf of the Association of Coloproctology of Great Britain and Ireland.
- Hartmann's procedure was found to be associated with a significantly higher complication rate, in-hospital mortality rate and length of hospital stay. However it was also demonstrated that Hartmann's procedure is significantly more likely to be

performed on profoundly unwell patients, by non-specialists and in the emergency setting.

- Having adjusting for case mix this study demonstrates that Hartmann's procedure may be independently associated with a higher risk of adverse outcome when compared with RPA.

References
1 Constantinides VA, Tekkis PP, Senapati A. Prospective multicentre evaluation of adverse outcomes following treatment for complicated diverticular disease. *Br J Surg.* 2006; **93**: 1503–13.
2 Banerjee S, Leather AJM, Rennie JA, *et al.* Feasibility and morbidity of reversal of Hartmann's. *Colorectal Dise.* 2005; **7**: 454–9.
3 Myers E, Hurley M, O'Sullivan GC, *et al.* Laparoscopic peritoneal lavage for generalized peritonitis due to perforated diverticulitis. *Br J Surg.* 2008; **95**: 97–101.
4 David GG, Al-Sarira AA, Willmott S, *et al.* Use of Hartmann's procedure in England. *Colorectal Dis.* 2008; **11**: 308–12.

4.4 Incision and drainage of a cutaneous abscess
Key points
An abscess is an accumulation of pus within an inflammatory capsule formed from adjacent tissues. Cutaneous abscesses can occur anywhere on the body, but common locations include the axillae, buttocks, breasts and limbs.

Although abscesses eventually discharge spontaneously, the purpose of surgery is to curtail symptoms and prevent fistulation and chronic or recurrent episodes of sepsis.

Procedural considerations
- Drainage is frequently performed under local anaesthetic. Local anaesthetic agents are thought to perform poorly in the acidic milieu of an abscess, therefore a general anaesthetic should be considered for large or deep lesions and in areas that are difficult to anaesthetise.
- The abscess is punctured at the point of maximum fluctuancy. If possible, the incision is extended along lines of natural skin tension. It should be sufficient to allow continued drainage and prevent early skin bridging. Loculations are broken

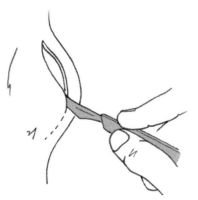

FIGURE 4.4 Drainage of abscess.

down digitally or with gentle instrumentation before the cavity is irrigated and packed loosely. Overpacking may cause increased pain and ischaemia. Healing is by secondary intention.[1]

Postoperative considerations
- Home same day or next.
- Daily dressing changes.
- Packed wounds take approximately 4–6 weeks to heal.

Additional considerations
- There is evidence that routine microbial cultures do not alter management or outcome, although they are advocated by some groups in order to identify local patterns of resistance and atypical microbes.[2]
- In the absence of cellulitis, the routine use of postoperative antibiotics is not indicated.[2]
- Traditionally, healing by secondary intention is advocated. Some studies suggest that primary closure improves outcome, but the literature is divided on this point and good quality prospective evidence is lacking.[2]
- The use of packing material is standard practice. However it is an empirical manoeuvre, which has not been substantially addressed in the literature. Similarly, the frequency with which dressings are changed is at the discretion of the practitioner and not founded on evidence.

CONSENT FORM
Name of procedure: Incision and drainage of cutaneous abscess
Benefits:
> Treatment of abscess
> Relieve symptoms
> Prevent fistula

Risks:
General:
> Bleeding
> Numbness
> Risks of LA/GA
> Scar

Specific:
> Cellulitis
> Delayed wound healing
> Recurrence

Procedure involves: Local or general anaesthesia

Key publications
Hankin AH, Everett WW. Are antibiotics necessary after incision and drainage of a cutaneous abscess? *Ann Emerg Med.* 2007; **6**: 232–4.[3]
- Review article: the search strategy uncovered three randomised trials spanning 30 years. This included a double-blind randomised controlled trial, the impact of which was limited by its size and the exclusion of patients with significant

co-morbidity. However, each trial concluded that patients treated with incision and drainage alone exhibit healing at the same rate as patients treated with supplementary antibiotics. None of the studies specifically addressed the issue of antibiotic use for abscesses with surrounding cellulitis.

Thirumalaikumar S, Kommu S. Best evidence topic reports: aspiration of breast abscesses. *Emerg Med J.* 2004; **21**: 333–4.[4]
- A review article including six studies of varying methodology. Overall the quality of the studies was poor. Only one study directly compared the use of aspiration with incision and drainage under local anaesthetic.
- The management of breast abscesses is subtly different to that of other cutaneous abscesses. Frequently, small abscesses, and abscesses in which the overlying skin is not immediately threatened, are treated by needle aspiration. This is often performed under ultrasound guidance and may be repeated if necessary.

References
1 Fitch MT, Manthey DE, McGinnis HD, *et al* Abscess incision and drainage. *N Engl J Med.* 2007; **357**: e20.
2 Korownyk C, Allan GM. Evidence-based approach to abscess management. *Can Fam Physician.* 2007; **53**: 1680–4.
3 Hankin AH, Everett WW. Are antibiotics necessary after incision and drainage of a cutaneous abscess? *Ann Emerg Med.* 2007; **6**: 232–4.
4 Thirumalaikumar S, Kommu S. Best evidence topic reports: aspiration of breast abscesses. *Emerg Med J.* 2004; **21**: 333–4.

4.5 Hernia repair: open inguinal hernia repair
Key points
Hernia is defined as the protrusion of all or part of an organ through the wall of the cavity in which it is contained. Inguinal hernias account for 75% of abdominal wall hernias.[1] They are described as direct or indirect depending on whether the hernia sac protrudes directly through the posterior wall of the inguinal canal or whether it passes indirectly into the canal via the deep inguinal ring.

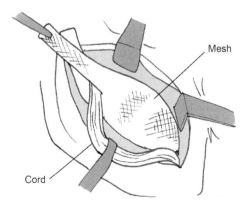

Mesh

Cord

FIGURE 4.5 Inguinal hernia repair.

The lifetime risk of an inguinal hernia is 27% for men and 3% for women. Open inguinal hernia repair can be achieved using a mesh technique (Lichtenstein repair) or a non-mesh technique (Shouldice repair).

Procedural considerations
- Day case.
- General/regional/local anaesthesia.
- The incision is placed 1 cm above and parallel to the inguinal ligament. It extends from the deep inguinal ring laterally to the pubic tubercle medially. The subcutaneous fat is divided to expose the external oblique aponeurosis which is opened along the axis of the inguinal canal to expose the cord structures beneath. The sac and the cord structures are defined before the sac is opened, ligated and returned to the abdominal cavity.
- The Lichtenstein repair differs from the Shouldice repair as a mesh is used to reinforce the posterior wall of the inguinal canal before the wound is closed in layers.

Postoperative considerations
- Immediate mobilisation with adequate analgesia.
- Simple dressing.

Additional considerations
Alternative options:
- Watchful waiting
  - This is acceptable for patients with minimal symptoms as incarceration and strangulation occurs only rarely.[2]
- Laparoscopic repair
  - There are two laparoscopic options: the transabdominal preperitoneal procedure (TAPP) and the totally extraperitoneal procedure (TEP). TAPP enables the reduction of the hernia via the peritoneal cavity. A mesh is inserted through the peritoneum and is anchored over the potential hernia site. TEP is achieved without entering the peritoneal cavity. The National Institute for Health and Clinical Excellence (NICE) recommends laparoscopic surgery as one of the treatment options for inguinal hernia repair. It recommends that patients should be informed of the risks and benefits of open and laparoscopic techniques, to enable them to choose between the procedures.

CONSENT FORM
Name of procedure: Primary inguinal hernia repair
Benefits:
    Treatment of symptoms
    Prevention of hernia incarceration and strangulation
Risks:
  Minor:[5,6]
    Haematoma: 6%–19%
    Seroma: 1.5%–2.2%
    Superficial wound infection: 0.5%–3.8%
    Persistent groin or testicular pain: 5.6%–10.8%
    Persistent numbness: 2%–4.2%

Major:
 Recurrence: 0.9%–2.1%[5,6]
 Testicular atrophy: 0.5%–2.5%[3,4]
 Vascular injury, visceral injury and deep mesh infections are rare.
Procedure involves: General/regional/local anaesthesia

Key publications

Scott N, Go PM, Graham P, et al. Open mesh versus non-mesh for groin hernia repair. Cochrane Database Syst Rev. 2001; 3: CD002197.[5]
- A systematic review of 20 trials comparing mesh and non-mesh techniques for groin hernia repair. No clear differences were identified in terms of major and minor complications between the two groups although there is a suggestion that persistent pain is less frequent after mesh repair.
- Fewer hernia recurrences were noted following mesh repair (Peto OR: 0.37, 95% CI: 0.26 to 0.51).

McCormack K, Scott N, Go PM, *et al.* EU Hernia Trialists Collaboration. Laparoscopic techniques versus open techniques for inguinal hernia repair. Cochrane Database Syst Rev. 2003; 1: CD001785.[6]
- A systematic review of 41 trials comparing laparoscopic and open inguinal hernia repair techniques. Operation times for laparoscopic repair were longer and there was a higher risk of rare serious complications. Return to usual activities was faster, and there was less persisting pain and numbness. Hernia recurrence was not significantly different to open mesh methods.

Wake BL, McCormack K, Fraser C, *et al.* Transabdominal preperitoneal (TAPP) vs. totally extraperitoneal (TEP) laparoscopic techniques for inguinal hernia repair. Cochrane Database Syst Rev. 2005; 1: CD004703.[7]
- A systematic review of randomised studies, quasi-randomised studies and case series, comparing two laparoscopic approaches for inguinal hernia repair. There is no clear difference between the two techniques in terms of length of hospital stay, haematoma, and return to normal activity. There is a suggestion that TAPP is associated with a higher rate of port site hernia and visceral injury, but there is insufficient data to draw firm conclusions.

References
1 Jenkins JT, O'Dwyer PJ. Inguinal hernias. *BMJ*. 2008; **336**: 269–72.
2 Fitzgibbons RJ Jr, Giobbie-Hurder A, Gibbs JO, *et al.* Watchful waiting in minimally symptomatic men: a randomised clinical trial. *JAMA*. 2006; **295**: 285–92.
3 Douek M, Smith G, Oshowo A, *et al.* Prospective randomised controlled trial of laparoscopic versus open inguinal hernia mesh repair: 5-year follow-up. *BMJ*. 2003; **326**: 1012–3.
4 Fitzgibbons RJ Jr. Can we be sure that polypropylene mesh causes infertility? *Ann Surg.* 2005; **241**: 559–61.
5 Scott N, Go PM, Graham P, *et al.* Open mesh versus non-mesh for groin hernia repair. Cochrane Database Syst Rev. 2001; 3: CD002197.
6 McCormack K, Scott N, Go PM, *et al.* EU Hernia Trialists Collaboration. Laparoscopic techniques versus open techniques for inguinal hernia repair. Cochrane Database Syst Rev. 2003; 1: CD001785.

7 Wake BL, McCormack K, Fraser C, *et al.* Transabdominal preperitoneal (TAPP) vs. totally extraperitoneal (TEP) laparoscopic techniques for inguinal hernia repair. Cochrane Database Syst Rev. 2005; 1: CD004703.

4.6 Pilonidal sinus excision

Key points
Pilonidal sinus disease usually manifests in the natal cleft of the sacrococcygeal area. The pathogenesis is uncertain, although the sinus tracts are likely to form as part of an inflammatory process within hair follicles. Their reported incidence is 26 per 100 000 of population with young males disproportionately affected.[1] In approximately 50% of cases, the index presentation is due to acute abscess formation[2] which is treated by incision and drainage. The treatment for those presenting with chronic pilonidal sinus disease is, however, far more contentious. Multiple surgical techniques are in current use (often within the same department), reflecting the lack of consensus on this point.

Procedural considerations
* The incidence of pilonidal sinus disease decreases through adulthood and there is a tendency to grow out of the disease. Furthermore, no single surgical option is entirely satisfactory. Careful selection of surgical technique is therefore essential and major surgery should be reserved for complex cases and recurrent disease. Although the optimal treatment for simple pilonidal disease is unclear, there appears to be some benefit in moving the healing point away from the midline cleft (so-called 'off-midline' techniques).[5] Whenever possible surgery should be performed in the day-case setting and under local anaesthesia.[3,4]
* Simple surgical options
    – Excision with healing by secondary intention.
    – Excision marsupialisation.
    – Excision with primary midline closure.
    – Excision with primary 'off-midline' closure (Bascom/Karydakis).

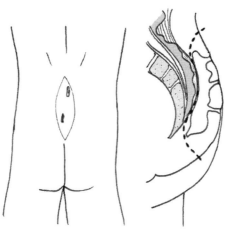

FIGURE 4.6 Pilonidal sinus excision.

Postoperative considerations
* Regular dressing changes until wound healing is achieved.
* Keep surgical field free of hair by shaving or other depilation methods.
* Avoid excessive walking or sitting in the early postoperative period.

Additional considerations
Other surgical options:
* Excision with flap reconstruction (Limberg/rhomboid/V-Y).
* Z-plasty.

CONSENT FORM
Name of procedure: Pilonidal sinus excision
Benefits:
    Treatment of pilonidal sinus
    Relief of symptoms
Risks.
  General:
    Bleeding/haematoma/seroma
    Risks of anaesthetic
  Specific:
    Infection:
      All primary closure techniques: 0%–23%, median 6%[5]
      Healing by secondary intention: 0%–30%, median 5%[5]
  Recurrence:
    All primary closure techniques: 0%–24%, median 9%[5]
    Healing by secondary intention: 0%–12.5%, median 4.5%[5]
Procedure involves: General/local anaesthesia

Key publications
McCallum I, King PM, Bruce J. Healing by primary closure versus open healing after surgery for pilonidal sinus: systematic review and meta-analysis. *BMJ*. 2008; **336**: 868–71.[5]
* Systematic review and meta-analyses of 18 randomised controlled trials.
* 12 trials compared open healing with various primary closure techniques. Six trials compared midline and off-midline (or asymmetric) primary closure. Flap reconstruction techniques were included in the off-midline group. More rapid healing was achieved with primary closure compared with open healing, with no significant difference in infection rate. Recurrence was less likely to occur with open healing (RR: 0.42, 95% CI: 0.26–0.66). However, some of the lowest infection and recurrence rates were achieved in off-midline or primary closure sub-groups. In comparison, midline closure is associated with higher infection rates (RR: 4.7, 95% CI: 1.93–11.45) and higher rates of recurrence (OR: 4.95, 95% CI: 2.18–11.24). The study concludes that off-midline closure should be the standard management when primary closure is the desired surgical option.

Bascom J. Surgical treatment of pilonidal disease. *BMJ*. 2008; **336**: 842–3.[6]
* An editorial exploring the balance between the severity of disease and the invasiveness of the surgical technique employed, tempering the fashion towards extensive excision in all cases. The author suggests that early primary disease can

be treated simply by the removal of hair and keratin from the pits of origin, whilst treatment of more advanced primary disease should involve abscess drainage through an off-midline incision and excision of midline pits (Bascom's procedure). Recurrent disease, extensive tissue involvement and the presence of multiple pits should be addressed by reducing the depth of the cleft and mobilising a flap to form an off-midline wound (Bascom's cleft lift procedure).

- Although the literature does not clearly demonstrate the superiority of Bascom's procedures over other techniques, the principle of tailoring the intervention to the individual circumstances is sound.

References

1 Sondenaa K, Nesvik I, Anderson E, *et al*. Patient characteristics and symptoms in chronic pilonidal sinus disease. *Int J Colorectal Dis*. 1995; **10**(1): 39–42.
2 Bascom J. Pilonidal disease: long-term results of follicle removal. *Dis Colon Rectum*. 1983; **26**: 800–7.
3 Naja MZ, Ziade MF, El Rajab M. Sacrococcygeal local anaesthesia versus general anaesthesia for pilonidal sinus surgery: a prospective randomised trial. *Anaesthesia*. 2003; **58**: 1007–12.
4 Abdul-Ghani AKM, Abdul-Ghani AN, Ingham Clark CL. Day-case surgery for pilonidal sinus. *Ann R Coll Surg Eng*. 2006; **88**: 656–8.
5 McCallum I, King PM, Bruce J. Healing by primary closure versus open healing after surgery for pilonidal sinus: systematic review and meta-analysis. *BMJ*. 2008; **336**: 868–71.
6 Bascom J. Surgical treatment of pilonidal disease. *BMJ*. 2008; **336**: 842–3.

4.7 Haemorrhoids: injection, banding or infrared coagulation

Key points

Haemorrhoids are abnormal swellings of the anal cushions present in the subepithelial space of the anal canal. These cushions contain direct arteriovenous communications between the terminal branches of the superior rectal arteries and the superior, inferior, and middle rectal veins. Their purpose is to aid continence.

Haemorrhoids are classified as internal or external depending on their position relative to the dentate line. 1st degree haemorrhoids are symptomatic but do not prolapse; 2nd degree haemorrhoids prolapse but reduce spontaneously; 3rd degree haemorrhoids require manual reduction and 4th degree haemorrhoids are irreducible.

Rubber band ligation (RBL) is performed for symptomatic 1st, 2nd and small 3rd degree haemorrhoids. It is a convenient first-line intervention as it can be performed in the outpatient setting and repeated if necessary.

Procedural considerations

- Performed in the outpatient setting.
- Anaesthesia is not required. The application of the band is painless as somatic sensory nerves are absent above the anal transition zone.
- RBL is achieved using a suction device to draw rectal mucosa and the blood vessels feeding the haemorrhoidal complex into a band applicator. The application should be at least 2 cm proximal to the dentate line to prevent pain. Up to three bands can be applied in a single session.

Postoperative considerations

- Patient advice leaflet.

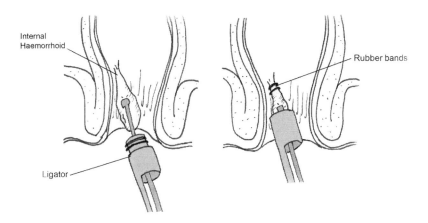

FIGURE 4.7 Rubber band ligation of haemorrhoids.

- Padding for underwear.
- Simple analgesia as required.

Additional considerations
Alternative procedures:
- The most established alternative outpatient intervention is injection sclerotherapy. This is easily performed via a proctoscope and involves the submucosal injection of a phenol-based sclerosant causing thrombosis of the haemorrhoidal vessels and sclerosis of overlying mucosa.
- Photocoagulation is another alternative and involves scarring haemorrhoidal tissue with pulses of infrared radiation from the tip of a probe.

CONSENT FORM

Name of procedure: Outpatient management of haemorrhoids – rubber band ligation

Benefits:
    Treatment of symptoms associated with haemorrhoids

Risks:
    Recurrence: 68% at 4 to 5 years[1]
    Minor complications:
        Mild pain: 5%–60%[1]
        Urinary retention, minor bleeding, ulceration of the rectal mucosa, painful haemorrhoidal thrombosis and perianal abscess: <5%[2]
    Major complications:
        Haemorrhage requiring readmission to hospital: 1.2%[2]
        Pelvic sepsis (extremely rare)

Key publications
MacRae HM, Temple LK, McLeod RS. A meta-analysis of hemorrhoidal treatments. *Semin C R Surg.* 2002; **13**: 77–83.[3]

- A meta-analysis of 23 studies comparing the use of RBL, sclerotherapy, photocoagulation, haemorrhoidectomy and manual dilatation in the treatment of 1st, 2nd and 3rd degree haemorrhoids.
- RBL was shown to be more effective than sclerotherapy and less likely to require additional treatment than both sclerotherapy and photocoagulation.
- RBL associated with a significantly greater incidence of post-procedural pain than both other modalities.

References
1 Madoff RD, Fleshman JW. American Gastroenterological Association technical review on the diagnosis and treatment of hemorrhoids. *Gastroenterology*. 2004; **126**: 1463–73.
2 Bat I, Melzer E, Koler M, *et al*. Complications of rubber band ligation of symptomatic internal haemorrhoids. *Dis Colon Rectum*. 1993; **36**: 287–90.
3 MacRae HM, Temple LK, McLeod RS. A meta-analysis of hemorrhoidal treatments. *Semin C R Surg*. 2002; **13**: 77–83.

4.8 Haemorrhoidectomy: operative
Key points
Haemorrhoids are abnormal swellings of the anal cushions present in the subepithelial space of the anal canal. These cushions contain direct arteriovenous communications between the terminal branches of the superior rectal arteries and the superior, inferior, and middle rectal veins. Their purpose is to aid continence.

Procedural considerations
- Surgical intervention is reserved for symptomatic 4th degree haemorrhoids and large symptomatic 3rd degree haemorrhoids, which have failed to respond to conservative management.
- Day-case procedure.
- General/regional anaesthesia. Many surgeons use local anaesthetic for additional pain relief and to help define the plane between haemorrhoid and internal sphincter.
- The Milligan–Morgan haemorrhoidectomy is one of a number of related operative approaches. Haemorrhoids classically sit in the left lateral, right anterior and right posterior positions. They are sequentially drawn out of the anal canal and encircled

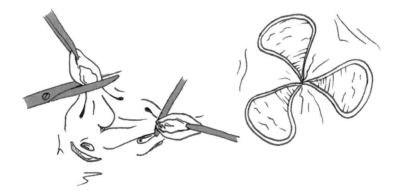

FIGURE 4.8 Haemorrhoidectomy.

by incisions extending to the anal verge on either side and to the internal sphincter beneath. Once the sphincter has been identified, the haemorrhoid is dissected from it to form a narrow pedicle which can then be ligated. The process repeated should create three haemorrhoidal beds separated by skin bridges in a three-leaf clover configuration. Wide skin bridges are essential if anal stenosis is to be avoided.

Postoperative considerations
- Dressing – no dressing/haemostatic pack or Voltarol suppository (surgeon's preference).
- Laxatives – Lactulose (early postoperative period), bulk laxatives (later if required).
- Metronidazole reduces postoperative pain.[1]

Additional considerations
Alternative treatments:
- The stapled haemorrhoidopexy (or anopexy) is less painful and permits a more rapid discharge and return to normal activity. The stapling device excises a proximal doughnut of mucosa, disrupting the blood supply to the haemorrhoid bed without forming a mucocutaneous defect in the anal canal. However it compares unfavourably in terms of symptom recurrence and reintervention for postoperative haemorrhage.[2]
- Ultrasound-guided haemorrhoidal artery ligation (HALO) – ultrasound-guided haemorrhoidal artery ligation is a relatively new procedure in which a purpose built Doppler probe is used to identify arteries supplying the haemorrhoidal bed in the submucosal plane. These vessels are suture ligated via a window in the head of the probe. The sutures are placed above the dentate line, so the procedure should be no more painful than band ligation. It qualifies as a minimally invasive procedure and is ideal for the day-case setting; no dissection is used and only light sedation is required. However long-term efficacy data is lacking.

CONSENT FORM

Name of procedure: Operative or Milligan–Morgan haemorrhoidectomy (MMH)

Benefits:
   Relief of symptoms (bleeding, palpable prolapse, pruritus)

Risks:
   Recurrence: at one year 4.3%[2]
   Minor complications:
      Minor postoperative bleeding is very common and can persist for several weeks.[3]
      Postoperative urinary retention (median 5%, range 0%–45%[3–9,10–13])
      Faecal impaction (median 4%, range 0%–14%[3–5,7,8,11,12,14])
      Anal fissure (median 4%, range 0%–6%[7,10,11,13–15])
      Anal stenosis (median 2.4%, range 0%–22%[4,7,10,11,13–16])
   Major complications:
      Continence issues
      Postoperative haemorrhage requiring reintervention <1 week – 3.2%[2]

Procedure involves: General/regional/local anaesthesia

Key publications

Shao WJ, Li GCH, Zhang ZHK, *et al.* Systematic review and meta-analysis of randomised controlled trials comparing stapled haemorrhoidopexy with conventional haemorrhoidectomy. *Br J Surg.* 2008; **95**: 147–60.[17]

- Meta-analysis of studies comparing stapled haemorrhoidopexy with conventional surgery – 29 randomised clinical trials – 2056 patients.
- Stapled haemorrhoidopexy required a shorter inpatient stay and operating time (p<0.001) and led to faster return to normal activity (p=0.017).
- There was no overall difference in terms of total complications between the two techniques but stapled haemorrhoidopexy was associated with a higher incidence of bleeding requiring reintervention (p=0.023) and a higher rate of recurrent disease (p<0.001).

Shalaby R, Desoky A. Randomised clinical trial of stapled vs. Milligan–Morgan haemorrhoidectomy. *Br J Surg.* 2001; **88**: 1049–53.[18]

- Largest randomised clinical trial with 100 patients in each arm followed up for 1 year following surgery – 20% attrition rate at 1 year.
- MMH group:
  - 3% incidence of anal fissure at 6 months – in each case the response to conservative management was adequate.
  - 6% incidence of anal stenosis at 12 months.
  - 2% incidence of bleeding requiring surgical intervention in the first two postoperative weeks.
  - 14% incidence of postoperative urinary retention.
- A number of studies have used anal manometry and mean incontinence scores to demonstrate that operative haemorrhoidectomy does not adversely affect continence.[3,7,15] Although adverse events are reported in the literature, the effect is mild or temporary and often refers to gas incontinence or discrimination issues. Soiling is exceptionally rare following MMH despite endoanal USS demonstrating sphincteric defects in up to 12% of patients following surgery.[16]

References

1 Carapeti EA, Kamm MA, McDonald PJ, *et al.* Double-blind randomised controlled trial of effect of metronidazole on pain after day-case haemorrhoidectomy. *Lancet.* 1998; **351**: 169–72.

2 Ho YK, Cheong WK, Tsang C, *et al.* Stapled hemorrhoidectomy – cost and effectiveness: randomized, controlled trial including incontinence scoring, anorectal manometry and endoanal ultrasound assessments at up to 3 months. *Dis Colon Rectum.* 2000; **43**: 1666–75.

3 Correa-Rovelo JM, Tellez O, Obregon L, *et al.* Stapled rectal mucosectomy vs. closed hemorrhoidectomy. *Dis Colon Rectum.* 2002; **45**: 1367–75.

4 Basdanis G, Papadopoulos VN, Michalopoulos A, *et al.* Randomized clinical trial of stapled hemorrhoidectomy vs. open with Ligasure for prolapsed piles. *Surg Endosc.* 2005; **19**: 235–9.

5 Chung CC, Cheung YS, Chan ESW, *et al.* Stapled hemorrhoidopexy vs. Harmonic Scalpel™ hemorrhoidectomy: a randomized trial. *Dis Colon Rectum.* 2005; **48**: 1213–9.

6 Racalbuto A, Aliotta I, Corsaro G, *et al.* Hemorrhoidal stapler prolapsectomy vs. Milligan–Morgan hemorrhoidectomy: a long-term randomized trial. *Int J Colorectal Dis.* 2004; **19**: 239–44.

7 Wilson MS, Pope V, Doran HE, *et al.* Objective comparison of stapled anopexy and open hemorrhoidectomy: a randomized, controlled trial. *Dis Colon Rectum.* 2002; **45**: 1437–44.

8 Cheetham MJ, Cohen CRG, Kamm MA, *et al.* A randomized, controlled trial of diathermy hemorrhoidectomy vs. stapled hemorrhoidectomy in an intended day-care setting with longer-term follow-up. *Dis Colon Rectum*. 2003; **46**: 491–7.

9 Khalil KH, O'Bichere A, Sellu D. Randomized clinical trial of sutured versus stapled closed haemorrhoidectomy. *Br J Surg*. 2000; **87**: 1352–5.

10 Ortiz H, Marzo J, Armendariz P. Randomized clinical trial of stapled haemorrhoidopexy versus conventional diathermy haemorrhoidectomy. *Br J Surg*. 2002; **89**: 1376–81.

11 Kraemer M, Parulava T, Roblick M, *et al.* Prospective randomized study: Proximate® PPH Stapler vs. LigaSure™ for hemorrhoidal surgery *Dis Colon Rectum*. 2005; **48**: 1517–22.

12 Gravie JF, Lehur PA, Huten N, *et al.* Stapled hemorrhoidopexy versus Milligan–Morgan hemorrhoidectomy: a prospective, randomized, multicenter trial with 2-year postoperative follow up. *Ann Surg*. 2005; **242**: 29–35.

13 Picchio M, Palimento D, Attanasio U, *et al.* Stapled vs. open hemorrhoidectomy: long-term outcome of a randomized controlled trial. *Int J Colorectal Dis*. 2006; **21**: 668–9.

14 Au-Yong I, Rowsell M, Hemingway DM. Randomised controlled clinical trial of stapled haemorrhoidectomy vs. conventional haemorrhoidectomy; a three-and-a-half year follow up. *Colorectal Dis*. 2004; **6**: 37–8.

15 Ganeo E, Altomare DF, Milito G, *et al.* Long-term outcome of a multicentre randomized clinical trial of stapled haemorrhoidopexy versus Milligan–Morgan haemorrhoidectomy. *Br J Surg*. 2007; **94**: 1033–7.

16 Felt-Bersma RJ, van Baren R, Koorevaar M, *et al.* Unsuspected sphincter defects shown by anal endosonography after anorectal surgery: a prospective study. *Dis Colon Rectum*. 1995; **38**: 249–53.

17 Shao WJ, Li GCH, Zhang ZHK, *et al.* Systematic review and meta-analysis of randomised controlled trials comparing stapled haemorrhoidopexy with conventional haemorrhoidectomy. *Br J Surg*. 2008; **95**: 147–60.

18 Shalaby R, Desoky A. Randomised clinical trial of stapled vs. Milligan–Morgan haemorrhoidectomy. *Br J Surg*. 2001; **88**: 1049–53.

4.9 Varicose vein surgery
Key points
Varicose veins (VV) are abnormally dilated and tortuous vessels predominantly caused by antegrade blood flow through incompetent valves. The aim of surgery is to reduce the pressure within these dilated superficial veins.

Procedural considerations
- Day-case procedure.
- General/regional anaesthesia.
- The groin incision overlies the saphenofemoral junction (SFJ) approximately 4 cm lateral to and 3 cm below the pubic tubercle. It is made in line with the skin crease, medial to the femoral pulse. This incision permits division of the tributaries of the long saphenous vein and flush ligation of the SFJ. A stripping device can then be manipulated along the course of the vein to the knee where it is retrieved via a small vertical incision. Stripping to the ankle is no longer performed due to the unacceptably high rate of saphenous nerve damage.
- Varicosities below the knee are marked preoperatively in indelible ink with the patient erect. They are retrieved via small stab incisions.

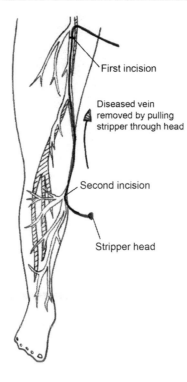

FIGURE 4.9 Varicose vein surgery.

Postoperative considerations
- Dressings: dry dressings, crepe bandages and an elastic support stocking. These are removed after 24 hours and replaced by grade 2 compression hosiery for two further weeks.
- Outpatient follow-up is not normally required.

Additional considerations
- Varicose veins are extremely common but rarely cause medical problems. Treatment is not essential; explanation and reassurance is often all that is indicated.
- Bleeding varicosities or skin ulceration resulting from varicose veins, carry the highest surgical priority. Superficial phlebitis, repetitive trauma, and aching varicosities carry lesser priority (the Vascular Society).
- Non-operative alternatives
  - Grade 2 compression hosiery reduces peripheral oedema and improves symptoms.
  - Sclerotherapy with agents such as sodium tetradecyl sulphate (STD) induces a chemical thrombophlebitis resulting in vein occlusion by fibrosis. Recanalisation and subsequent recurrence is common and the consensus is drifting towards its use as a second- or third-line therapy only.
- Minimally invasive surgery
  - There are two endovenous surgical options –radiofrequency ablation (VNUS™) and endovenous laser therapy (EVLT). Endovenous surgery can be performed

under local anaesthetic in a day-case or even outpatient setting. Patients with particularly tortuous or superficial veins are usually excluded due to the concomitant risk of thermal burns and skin hyperpigmentation. The results of minimally invasive techniques compare favourably with conventional surgery but are unlikely to obviate it. Furthermore, long-term follow-up data is lacking.

CONSENT FORM

Name of procedure: Varicose vein surgery – long saphenous vein ligation +/– multiple phlebectomies

Benefits:
Relief of symptoms

Risks:
Minor complications:
Bruising is a universal consequence of VV surgery, especially following phlebectomy.
Patients can expect residual bruising for up to 6 weeks.[5]
Bleeding
Wound infection or haematoma: 3%–14%[1,2,3]
Minor neurological disturbance – paraesthesia, dysaesthesia, numbness: 7%–27%[1,4]
Recurrent or residual VV (21%–37% between 2–5 years[8]). At 10 years up to 77% of patients will claim that their symptoms remain cured or much improved although 70% will have visible VV on the operated limb.[9]
Permanent skin discoloration – rare
Lymphatic leakage – rare
Major complications:
DVT: 0.5%–5.3%
PE: 0.17%[1,6]
Major vessel injury – common femoral artery or vein: 0.013%[7]

Procedure involves: General and/or regional anaesthesia

Key publications

Goodwin H. Litigation and surgical practice in the UK. *Br J Surg.* 2000; **87**: 977–9.[10]
- Varicose vein surgery is the most frequent source of litigation in general surgery. The most common reason for compensation is damage to associated structures, which includes causing minor neurological disturbances. However, claims rarely arise from a single issue, and communication failure at the time of consent is frequently a contributory factor.

Campbell B. Varicose veins and their management. *BMJ.* 2006; **333**: 287–92.[11]
- An excellent clinical review, summarising the pathophysiology and clinical manifestation of VVs. The available treatment modalities are explored in detail.

References

1 Critchley G, Handa A, Maw A, *et al.* Complications of varicose vein surgery. *Ann R Coll Surg Eng.* 1997; **79**: 105–10.
2 Corder AP, Schache DJ, Farquharson SM, *et al.* Wound infection following high saphenous ligation: a trial comparing two skin closure techniques, subcuticular polyglycolic

acid and interrupted monofilament nylon mattress sutures. *J R Coll Surg Edinb*. 1991; **36**: 100–2.

3 Defty C, Eardley N, Taylor M, *et al*. A comparison of the complication rates following unilateral and bilateral varicose vein surgery. *Eur J Vasc Endovasc Surg*. 2008; **35**: 745–9.
4 Wood JJ, Chant H, Langharne M, *et al*. A prospective study of cutaneous nerve injury following long saphenous vein surgery. *Eur J Vasc Endovasc Surg*. 2005; **30**: 654–8.
5 Subramonia S, Lees TA. Sensory abnormalities and bruising after long saphenous vein stripping: impact on short-term quality of life. *J Vasc Surg*. 2005; **42**: 510–14.
6 Van Rij AM, Chai J, Hill GB, *et al*. Incidence of deep vein thrombosis after varicose vein surgery. *Br J Surg*. 2004; **91**: 1582–5.
7 Frings N, Glowacki P, Kohajda J. Major vascular and neural injuries in varicose vein surgery: prospective registration of the complication rate in long and short saphenous vein operation [German]. *Chirurg*. 2001; **72**: 1032–5.
8 Beale RJ, Gough MJ. Treatment options for primary varicose veins: a review. *Eur J Vasc Endovasc Surg*. 2005; **30**: 83–95.
9 Campbell WB, Vijay Kumar A, Collin TW, *et al*. The outcome of varicose vein surgery at 10 years: clinical findings, symptoms and patient satisfaction. *Ann R Coll Surg Engl*. 2003; **85**: 52–7.
10 Goodwin H. Litigation and surgical practice in the UK. *Br J Surg*. 2000; **87**: 977–9.
11 Campbell B. Varicose veins and their management. *BMJ*. 2006; **333**: 287–92

4.10 Major lower limb amputation
Key points
Peripheral arterial occlusive disease accounts for the majority of lower limb amputations in the UK. Amputation is considered when revascularisation is not possible or has been unsuccessful. Amputation can be a life-saving manoeuvre in the presence of widespread infection or necrosis and frequently provides symptomatic relief, improved quality of life and improved function.

Procedural considerations:
- General/spinal anaesthesia.
- Typically transfemoral amputations are fashioned with equally sized anterior and posterior myocutaneous flaps.

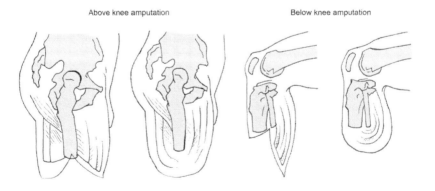

FIGURE 4.10 Above- and below-knee amputations.

- Transtibial amputations are traditionally performed using a long posterior (Burgess) flap.
- Some surgeons prefer skew flaps as they are fashioned on recognised vascular pedicles based around the long and short saphenous veins. However, skew flaps do not confer any advantage over the more established posterior flap technique.[1]
- The Gritti–Stokes' technique is a through-knee amputation.

Postoperative considerations:
- Multidisciplinary management – surgeons, rehabilitation team (physiotherapists, occupational therapy), counselling, prosthetics department, pain team.
- Tight fitting stump dressing should be avoided initially. Once the stump has healed, graduated pressure dressings such as the Juzo stocking can be used to shape the stump and reduce oedema.

Additional considerations
- The level at which an amputation is performed is determined by the distal extent of well-vascularised, sensate tissue. However, the amputation level is also influenced by the patient's rehabilitation potential.
- If walking with a prosthetic limb is a realistic aim, a functioning knee joint should be preserved whenever possible. However, if there is a greater than 35° flexion contracture of the knee then a transfemoral amputation may provide a better functional outcome.
- If the patient is likely to be wheelchair or bed bound, the Gritti–Stokes' knee disarticulation is usually employed as it provides the longest possible lever for transferring and balanced sitting, without the risk of a disabling flexion contracture of the knee.

CONSENT FORM
Name of procedure: Major lower limb amputation – above-knee/below-knee amputation (AKA/BKA)

Benefits:
    Amputate infected, necrotic tissue
    Save life
    Improve function and quality of life

Risks:
    General:[2]
        Myocardial infarction: 1.9%
        Congestive Cardiac Failure: 3.8%
        Pneumonia: 3%
        Acute Renal Failure: 2.1%
        CVA: 0.5%
        30-day mortality 7.4%: AKA 17.3%, BKA 4.2%[2]

    Specific:
        Phantom sensations: 53.1%–100%[3]
        Stump pain: 6%–76.1%[3]
        Phantom limb pain: 50%–79.6%[3]
        Wound infection: 7%–26.4%[4,5]
        Healing issues (non-healing, delayed healing, dehiscence, necrosis)
        Neuroma

Procedure involves: General/regional/local anaesthesia

Key publications

Subramaniam B, Pomposelli F, Talmor D, *et al*. Perioperative and long-term morbidity and mortality after above-knee and below-knee amputations in diabetics and nondiabetics. *Anesth Analg*. 2005; **100**: 1241–7.[2]
* Retrospective review of 954 patients undergoing major lower limb amputations for dysvascularity.
* 30-day mortality 7.4% overall. Positive predictive factors of inpatient mortality were renal insufficiency (OR=2.15, p=0.019), and amputation level – AKA>BKA (OR=4.35, p<0.001).
* Diabetes was not a significant predictor of 30-day in-patient mortality.
* 10-year survival following AKA=19% and BKA=28.5%.

Sanam K, Neumann V, O'Connor R, *et al*. Predicting walking ability following lower limb amputation: a systematic review of the literature. *J Rehabil Med*. 2009; **41**: 593–603.[6]
* Systematic review of 57 studies exploring the factors that predict walking ability following lower limb amputation.
* Unilateral surgery, distal amputation level, and younger age are predictive of better walking ability. Cognitive function, delay between amputation and rehabilitation and preoperative mobility also have predictive value.

References
1 Tisi PV, Callam MJ. Type of incision for below-knee amputation. Cochrane Database Syst Rev. 2004; 1: CD003749.
2 Subramaniam B, Pomposelli F, Talmor D, *et al*. Perioperative and long-term morbidity and mortality after above-knee and below-knee amputations in diabetics and nondiabetics. *Anesth Analg*. 2005; **100**: 1241–7.
3 Richardson C, Glenn S, Horgan M. Incidence of phantom phenomena including phantom limb pain 6 months after major lower limb amputation in patients with peripheral vascular disease. *Clin J Pain*. 2006; **22**: 353–8.
4 Lim TS, Finlayson A, Thorpe JM, *et al*. Outcomes of a contemporary amputation series. *Aust N Z J Surg*. 2006; **76**: 300–5.
5 Ploeg AJ, Lardenoye JW, Vracken Peeters MP, *et al*. Contemporary series of morbidity and mortality after lower limb amputation. *Eur J Vasc Endovasc Surg*. 2005; **29**: 633–7.
6 Sanam K, Neumann V, O'Connor R, *et al*. Predicting walking ability following lower limb amputation: a systematic review of the literature. *J Rehabil Med*. 2009; **41**: 593–603.

5

Neurosurgery

5.1 Insertion of an intracranial pressure monitor
Key points
Intracranial pressure (ICP) monitoring uses a pressure monitor placed inside the skull and dura mater to measure and record intracranial pressure.

Procedural considerations
- General or local anaesthetic. IV antibiotics.
- Position: patient is supine with head in a neutral position.
- Site: Kocher's point (coronal) places the catheter in the frontal horn. If no clinical indications, the non-dominant hemisphere (right side) is selected.
- Entry site: 2–3 cm from the midline in the mid-pupillary line and 1 cm anterior to the coronal suture.
- The cranial access kit and the Camino bolt is opened in a sterile fashion.
- Stab incision is performed over the planned burr hole site.
- A twist drill hole is placed through skull without penetrating the dura. The safety nut on the drill is used to prevent plunging. The bolt is screwed into the skull until finger tight.
- The dura is opened with a probe (available in the cranial access kit).
- The catheter is directed perpendicular to the brain's surface to a depth of 5–7 cm and the presence of a waveform is confirmed.
- The bolt is tightened around the catheter to secure in place.

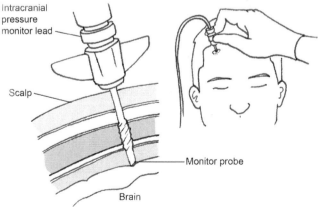

FIGURE 5.1 Intracranial pressure monitor.

Additional considerations

Contraindications:

- Coagulopathy.

CONSENT FORM

Name of procedure: Insertion of an intracranial pressure (ICP) monitor

Benefits:

    To diagnose, monitor and treat raised intracranial pressure

    Monitor cerebral perfusion pressure

    {Cerebral perfusion pressure = mean arterial pressure (MAP) – intracranial pressure (ICP)}

Risks:

  General:

    Headache[1]

    Bleeding (2.8%). The risk of significant haematoma requiring surgical evacuation is 0.5%[2]

    Infection 14%[3]

  Specific:

    Cerebrospinal fluid (CSF) leakage

    Inaccurate recordings

    Misplacement

    Malfunction or obstruction

Procedure involves: General anaesthesia/local anaesthesia

Key publications

Saul TG, Ducker TB. Effect of intracranial pressure monitoring and aggressive treatment on mortality in severe head injury. *J Neurosurg.* 1982; **56**: 498–503.[4]

- This study compared two groups of patients (total 233) with severe head injuries who underwent ICP monitoring.
- All patients had a GCS ≤7 and all received similar initial treatment.
- The overall mortality between the two groups was 46% and 28%, respectively.
- The study reconfirmed the high mortality rate if ICP was ≥25 mmHg.
- Data suggested that early aggressive treatment based on ICP monitoring, significantly reduced the incidence of ICP of ≥25 mmHg and the overall mortality rate from severe head injury.

Juul N, Morris GF, Marshall SB, *et al*. Intracranial hypertension and cerebral perfusion pressure: Influence on neurological deterioration and outcome in severe head injury. *J Neurosurg.* 2000; **92**(1): 1–6.[5]

- Prospective international multicentre randomised double-blind trial.
- 427 patients evaluated.
- Treatment protocols for the management of severe head injury should emphasise the immediate reduction of raised ICP to less than 20 mmHg.
- CPP >60 mmHg appeared to have little influence on the outcome of patients with severe head injuries.

References

1 Bullock R, Chesnut R, Clifton G et al. Guidelines for the management of severe head

injury. Brain Trauma Foundation American Association of Neurological Surgeons Joint Section on Neurotrauma and Critical Care. *J Neurotrauma* 1996; **13**: 641–734.

2 Bullock R, Chesnut RM, Clifton G, Ghajar J, Marion DW, Narayan RK, *et al.*: Guidelines for the management of severe traumatic brain injury. Brain Trauma Foundation. *J Neurotrauma* 2000; **17**: 449–554.

3 Narayan RK, Kishore PR, Becker DP, *et al.* Intracranial pressure – to monitor or not to monitor: a review of our experience with severe head injuries. *J Neurosurg.* 1982; **56**: 650–9.

4 Saul TG, Ducker TB. Effect of intracranial pressure monitoring and aggressive treatment on mortality in severe head injury. *J Neurosurg.* 1982; **56**: 498–503.

5 Juul N, Morris GF, Marshall SB, *et al.* Intracranial hypertension and cerebral perfusion pressure: Influence on neurological deterioration and outcome in severe head injury. *J Neurosurg.* 2000; **92**(1): 1–6.

5.2 Insertion of an external ventricular drain

Key points

The insertion of an extraventricular drain (EVD) allows for the temporary drainage of cerebrospinal fluid (CSF) from the ventricles of the brain in order to treat raised intracranial pressure and hydrocephalus when the normal flow of CSF is obstructed.

Procedural considerations

- General, regional or local anaesthetic. IV antibiotics.
- Position: patient is supine with head in neutral position.
- Site: Kocher's point (coronal) places the catheter in the frontal horn. If no clinical indications, select the non-dominant hemisphere (right side).
- Entry site: 2–3 cm from midline in the mid-pupillary line and 1 cm anterior to the coronal suture.
- Burr hole created by holding the perforator perpendicular to the skull.
- Dura is opened. Bipolar cautery is used to coagulate the dural edges.

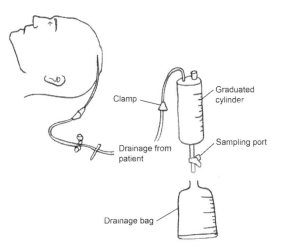

FIGURE 5.2 Insertion of an external ventricular drain.

- A ventricular catheter is inserted perpendicular to the brain surface to a depth of 5–6 cm. Aim towards the ipsilateral medial canthus.
- The stylet is withdrawn from the catheter to check for CSF flow. Measure opening pressure.
- A tunnelling device is attached to the distal end of the catheter. Stabilise the catheter at the burr hole, tunnel the distal portion under the galea aponeurosis to a skin exit site at least 5 cm away from the entry point.
- CSF drainage is reconfirmed.
- The galea aponeurosis is closed with 2.0 vicryl and apply skin clips.
- The catheter is secured to the scalp with a U-stitch with 3.0 nylon. The distal end of the catheter is connected to a drainage system.

Postoperative considerations
- CSF is sent for analysis (biochemistry, bacteriology +/– cytology).

CONSENT FORM
Name of procedure: Insertion of an external ventricular drain (ventriculostomy)
Benefits:
 To measure intracranial pressure (ICP)
 To treat raised ICP by drainage of cerebrospinal fluid (CSF)
 To treat CSF infection (administer intrathecal antibiotics)
 To allow for intraoperative brain relaxation to access deep brain structures
  and minimise brain retraction.
Risks:
 General:
  Infection 10%–17%[1,2,3]
  Bleeding 1%[1]
 Specific:
  CSF leakage
  Malposition requiring operative repositioning
  Malfunction, migration or blockage 6%[1]
  Aneurysm rupture (if the patient has an underlying cerebral aneurysm)[4]
Procedure involves: General/regional/local anaesthesia

Additional considerations
Contraindications:
- Coagulopathy or patients on anticoagulation (e.g. heparin, warfarin, aspirin).
- Vascular malformation or other mass lesions in the pathway of the catheter.

Key publications
Holloway KL, Barnes T, Choi S, *et al.* Ventriculostomy infections: the effect of monitoring duration and catheter exchange in 584 patients. *J Neurosurg.* 1996; **85**(3): 419–24.[2]
- 584 severely head-injured patients with ventriculostomies were prospectively collected.
- This study showed a relationship between ventriculitis and monitoring duration, but it was not simple or linear.
- There is a rising risk of infection over the first 10 days, but infection then becomes very unlikely despite a population that continues to be at risk.

- Patients whose catheters were replaced prior to 5 days did not have lower infection rates than those whose catheters were exchanged at more than 5-day intervals.
- Recommendation: catheters should be removed as quickly as possible; in circumstances in which prolonged monitoring is required, there was no benefit from catheter exchange.

Chan KH, Mann KS. Prolonged therapeutic external ventricular drainage: a prospective study. *Neurosurgery*. 1998; **23**: 436–8.[5]
- Over 2.5 years, therapeutic external ventricular drainage with a valve-regulated system was inserted.
- The mean duration of drainage was 16 days.
- All patients remained free from complications after 6 months. The system proved to be safe and reliable in patients requiring prolonged ventricular drainage.

References
1 Bullock RM, Chesnut RM, Clifton GL et al. Guidelines for the management of severe traumatic brain injury. *J Neuro trauma* 2000, **17**: 449–554.
2 Holloway KL, Barners T, Choi S, *et al.* Ventriculostomy infections: the effect of monitoring duration and catheter exchange in 584 patients. *J Neurosurg*. 1996; **85**: 419–24.
3 Lozier AP, Sciacca RR, Romagnoli MF, *et al.* Ventriculostomy-related infections: a critical review of the literature. *Neurosurg*. 2002; **51**: 170–82.
4 Voldby B, Enevoldsen EM. Intracranial pressure changes following aneurysm rupture: recurrent hemorrhage. *J Neurosurg*. 1982; **56**: 784–9.
5 Chan KH, Mann KS. Prolonged therapeutic external ventricular drainage: a prospective study. *Neurosurgery*. 1998; **23**: 436–8.

5.3 Insertion of a ventriculoperitoneal shunt
Key points
Insertion of a ventriculoperitoneal (VP) shunt is performed to relieve raised intracranial pressure. Cerebrospinal fluid is shunted from the lateral ventricle of the brain into the abdominal (peritoneal) cavity.

Procedural considerations
- General anaesthetic. IV antibiotics at induction.
- Position: patient is supine with head turned 90° to the opposite side with ipsilateral shoulder roll in place.
- Site: if no clinical indications, the non-dominant hemisphere (right side) is selected.
- Scalp incision: small semilunar scalp flap or linear incision.
- Frontal approach
  - Kocher's point (coronal) places the catheter in the frontal horn. Entry site: 2–3 cm from the midline in the mid-pupillary line and 1 cm anterior to the coronal suture.
- Occipital-parietal approach
  - Frazier burr hole: 3–4 cm from the midline, 6–7 cm above the inion.
  - Parietal boss: flat portion of the parietal bone.
  - 3 cm above and 3 cm posterior to the top of the pinna.
- Burr hole
  - Retractors pulled caudally in order for the burr hole to be placed 1 cm below the incision to ensure that no hardware lies under the suture line. The burr hole is created by holding the perforator perpendicular to the skull.

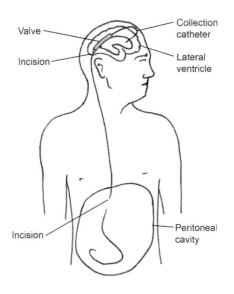

FIGURE 5.3 Ventriculoperitoneal shunt.

- Dural opening
  - Bipolar cautery is used to coagulate the dural edges.
- Abdominal entry
  - A horizontal incision is created 2 cm lateral and 2 cm superior to the umbilicus. The anterior rectus sheath is incised. Rectus muscle is split in layers. Long clamps placed on posterior rectus sheath and then incised. Additional clamps are placed on the peritoneum.
- The shunt is tunnelled from the scalp to the abdominal incision by inserting a metal trocar/passer in which the shunt is then passed.
- The ventricles are cannulated
  - The ventricular catheter is inserted perpendicular to the brain surface.
  - Frontal approach: the catheter is inserted to a depth of 5–6 cm. Aim towards the ipsilateral medial canthus.
  - Occipital-parietal approach: the catheter is inserted to a depth of 3 cm.
  - The stylet is withdrawn from the catheter to ensure CSF flow and to measure the opening pressure.
- Shunt assembly
  - Connect the valve between proximal and distal catheter. Secure with a silk tie.
- Assessment of catheter placement
  - Spontaneous CSF flow from distal end.
  - 10 mL of CSF is gently aspirated from the distal catheter with a blunt needle.
  - The shunt valve is easily pumped.
- Placement of peritoneal catheter
  - The shunt is placed in the peritoneal cavity.

Postoperative considerations
- CSF is sent for analysis (biochemistry, bacteriology +/– cytology).
- Neurological observations.

- Allow the patient to eat when bowel sounds are noted (due to an ileus).
- Shunt radiological series (AP and lateral skull, chest/abdominal X-rays).

Additional considerations

Contraindications:
- Necrotising enterocolitis.
- Recurrent peritonitis.
- Cerebrospinal fluid (CSF) infection.
- Coagulopathy.

CONSENT FORM

Name of procedure: Insertion of a ventriculoperitoneal shunt
Benefits:
    Treatment of:
        Communicating hydrocephalus
        Obstructive hydrocephalus, if a third ventriculostomy is contraindicated
          or failed
        Normal pressure hydrocephalus
        Symptomatic pseudotumour cerebri, if optic sheath fenestration and lum-
          boperitoneal shunting failed
    Revision of a malfunctioning shunt
Risks:
    Perioperative:
        Aberrant pass of ventricular catheter – too far or misdirected
        Intracerebral haemorrhage or intraventricular haemorrhage
        Injury to the abdominal viscera
        Pneumothorax
        Cervical spine injury from excessive head turning in predisposed patients
    Postoperative:
        Shunt malfunction and obstruction 12%–34%[1]
        Shunt infection, ventriculitis and peritonitis
        Over-shunting[2]
        Peritoneal catheter migration[3]
        Skin erosion
        Hydrocoele, peritoneal pseudocyst and ascites[4]
        Inguinal hernias (inserted while the processus vaginalis is patent)[5]
        Seizures – 5.5% risk of seizures in the first year after placement of a shunt,
          which drops to 1.1% after the 3rd year.[6]
Procedure involves: General anaesthesia

Key publications

Barnes NP, Jones SJ, Hayward RD, *et al.* Ventriculoperitoneal shunt block: what are the best predictive clinical indicators? *Arch Dis Child.* 2002; **87**(3): 198–201.[7]
- Prospective study.
- 53 patient referrals with a presumed diagnosis of shunt malfunction.
- Referral pattern, presenting symptoms/signs, CT scan results, operative findings and clinical outcome were recorded.

- Two groups were defined: (1) proven shunt block and (2) presumed normal shunt function.
- Common presenting features: headache, drowsiness and vomiting; 37 had operatively proven shunt malfunction, of whom 34 had shunt block and 3 shunt infection; 84% with shunt block had increased ventricle size when compared with previous imaging.
- Drowsiness was by far the best clinical predictor of VP shunt block. Headache and vomiting were less predictive of acute shunt blockage. When possible, CT scans should be compared to previous imaging. Not all cases of proven shunt blockage present with increased ventricle size.

References

1 Cozzens JW, Chandler JP. Increased risk of distal ventriculoperitoneal shunt obstruction associated with slit valves or distal slits in peritoneal catheter. *J Neurosurg.* 1997; **87**: 682–6.
2 Pudenz RH, Foltz EL. Hydrocephalus – overdrainage by ventricular shunts: a review and recommendations. *Surg Neurol.* 1991; **35**: 200–12.
3 Rush DS, Walsh JW. Abdominal complications of CSF–peritoneal shunts. *Monogr Neural Sci.* 1982; **8**: 52–4.
4 Bryant MS, Bremer AM, Tepas JJ, *et al.* Abdominal complications of ventriculoperitoneal shunts. *Am Surg.* 1988; **54**: 50–5.
5 Moazam F, Glenn JD, Kaplan BJ, *et al.* Inguinal hernias after ventriculoperitoneal shunt procedures in paediatric patients. *Surg Gynecol Obstet.* 1984; **159**: 570–2.
6 Dan N, Wade MJ. The incidence of epilepsy after ventricular shunting procedures. *J Neurosurg.* 1986; **65**: 19–21.
7 Barnes NP, Jones SJ, Hayward RD, *et al.* Ventriculoperitoneal shunt block: what are the best predictive clinical indicators? *Arch Dis Child.* 2002; **87**(3): 198–201.

Technical notes:

Ghajar J. A guide for ventricular catheter placement: technical note. *J Neurosurg.* 1985; **63**: 985–6.
Keskil S, Ceviker N, Baykaner K, *et al.* Index for optimum ventricular catheter length: technical note. *J Neurosurg.* 1991; **75**: 152–3.

5.4 Burr hole evacuation of a subdural haematoma
Key points
A subdural haematoma is a collection of blood formed between the dura mater and the arachnoid layer, secondary to tearing of a bridging vein and usually a result of head trauma. The chronic phase of a subdural haematoma begins several weeks after the event.

Procedural considerations
- General, regional or local anaesthetic. IV antibiotics at induction.
- Position: patient is supine with head in a neutral position.
- Transverse linear incision approximately 3 cm in length and positioned over the frontal and parietal convexities depending upon the extent and location of the chronic subdural haematoma.
- Burr hole: 2 cm diameter, frontal +/– parietal burr hole is made with a perforator.
- Dural opening: bipolar cautery is used to coagulate the dura, which is then opened with a cruciate incision. The dural leaflets are shrunk with additional cautery.
- Evacuation: following the spontaneous drainage of the chronic subdural

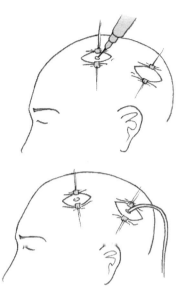

FIGURE 5.4 Chronic subdural haematoma evacuation.

haematoma, copious warm irrigation is used to remove any remaining haematoma. Irrigation continues until the fluid remains clear.
- Drain insertion: if required, a Jackson–Pratt drain is brought through the skin via a separate stab incision and inserted into the subdural space. The use of a subdural drain is associated with decreased rates of repeat surgery.
- Closure: bone wax is applied to the burr hole; the galea aponeurosis and skin is closed. If drain is inserted, a U-stitch is placed at the exit site and secured with a silk suture. A dressing is applied to the surgical wound.

Postoperative considerations
- The patient should remain in bed for the next 12–24 hours and then gently mobilised.

Additional considerations
Contraindications:
- Coagulopathy.
- Patients on anticoagulation (e.g. heparin, warfarin, aspirin).

CONSENT FORM
Name of procedure: Burr hole evacuation of a chronic subdural haematoma
Benefits:
> To evacuate:
>> A symptomatic subdural haematoma (e.g. headache, focal deficits, change in mental status)
>> A subdural haematoma with maximum thickness ≥1 cm, midline shift or mass effect

Risks:
 General:
  Infection (e.g. wound, subdural empyema and meningitis)[4]
  Seizures
 Specific:
 Perioperative:
  Inadequate removal of a chronic subdural haematoma
  Injury to the brain or laceration of the cortical vessels (bleeding)
 Postoperative:
  Persistence or recurrence of a subdural haematoma[1] – may result in failure
   of the brain to re-expand or re-accumulation of subdural fluid.
  Neurological deterioration 4%[2]
  Intracerebral haemorrhage 7%–5%[3]
  Pneumocephalus
 Procedure involves: General/regional/local anaesthesia

Key publications

Robinson RG. Chronic subdural hematoma: surgical management in 133 patients. *J Neurosurg.* 1984; **61**(2): 263–8.[5]
- Retrospective study.
- 133 patients with chronic subdural hematomas were treated surgically.
- The patients, aged 5–84 years, were graded according to the Bender scale.
- There were 107 unilateral and 26 bilateral haematomas.
- The clots were removed via burr holes without drainage.
- The high-risk groups were Bender grades 3–4, bilateral haematomas and the elderly.
- Patients appeared to benefit from brain inflation and lumbar injections for the treatment of intracranial hypotension.

Lind CR, Lind CJ, Mee EW. Reduction in the number of repeated operations for the treatment of subacute and chronic subdural hematomas by placement of subdural drains. *J Neurosurg.* 2003; **99**(1): 44–6.[6]
- 500 consecutive operations were performed for the treatment of subdural haematomas via burr holes.
- Rates of repeated surgery were compared in patients with and without subdural drains.
- Repeated operations were performed less frequently in patients who underwent subdural drain insertions.
- If technically feasible, subdural drains were recommended to be inserted regardless of brain expansion during surgery.

Santarius T, Kirkpatrick PJ, Ganesan D, *et al.* Use of drains versus no drains after burr-hole evacuation of chronic subdural haematoma: a randomised controlled trial. *Lancet.* 2009; **374**: 1067–73.[7]
- Randomised controlled trial.
- The aim of this study was to investigate the effect of drains on recurrence rates and clinical outcome.
- 269 patients with a chronic subdural haematoma for burr-hole drainage were assessed for eligibility.

- 108 patients were randomly assigned by block randomisation to receive a subdural drain and 107 patients were selected for no drain insertion.
- Primary endpoint was recurrence requiring re-drainage.
- The trial was stopped early because of the significant benefit in the reduction of recurrence.
- Use of a drain after burr-hole drainage of chronic subdural haematoma was safe and associated with reduced recurrence and mortality at 6 months.

References

1 Markwalder TM, Steinsiepe KF, Rohner M, *et al*. The course of chronic subdural hematomas after burr-hole craniostomy and closed-system drainage. *J Neurosurg*. 1981; **55**: 390–36.
2 Ernestus RI, Beldzinski P, Lanfermann H, *et al*. Chronic subdural hematomas: surgical treatment and outcome in 104 patients. *Surg Neurol*. 1997; **48**: 220–5.
3 Ogasawara K, Koshu K, Yoshimoto T, *et al*. Transient hyperaemia immediately after rapid decompression of chronic subdural haematoma. *Neurosurgery*. 1999; **45**: 484–9.
4 Dill SR, Cobbs CG, McDonald CK, Subdural empyema: analysis of 32 cases and review. *Clin Inf Dis*. 1995; **20**: 372–86.
5 Robinson RG. Chronic subdural hematoma: surgical management in 133 patients. *J Neurosurg*. 1984; **61**(2): 263–8
6 Lind CR, Lind CJ, Mee EW. Reduction in the number of repeated operations for the treatment of subacute and chronic subdural hematomas by placement of subdural drains. *J Neurosurg*. 2003; **99**(1): 44–6
7 Santarius T, Kirkpatrick PJ, Ganesan D, *et al*. Use of drains versus no drains after burr-hole evacuation of chronic subdural haematoma: a randomised controlled trial. *Lancet*. 2009; **374**: 1067–73.

5.5 Lumbar puncture

Key points
Removal of cerebrospinal fluid from the subarachnoid space in the lumbar region of the spinal cord for diagnostic or therapeutic purposes.

Procedural considerations
- General, regional or local anaesthetic.
- Lateral decubitus position (the patient's knees are drawn up to their stomach and their head is flexed to their chest) with the spine parallel to and at the edge of the bed; thereby flexing the vertebral column and widening the intervertebral space.
- The spinal cord terminates at the L1–2 level in adults and at the L2–3 level in children. A lumbar puncture should be performed at the L3–4 or L4–5 interspace.
- The L3–L4 interspace is located along the supracristal line (an imaginary line between the iliac crests) and the puncture site marked.
- Standard preparation and drape.
- The spinal needle is advanced through the skin, supraspinous ligament, interspinous ligament, ligamentum flavum, epidural space, dura and subarachnoid membrane into the subarachnoid space.
- A 'give' is felt when puncturing the ligamentum flavum and a loss of resistance will be noted when dura is penetrated.
- Once a CSF flashback is seen, the stylet is removed, the manometer is attached and the opening pressure measured (when the patient's legs are straightened).
- The needle is withdrawn and a dry sterile dressing applied.

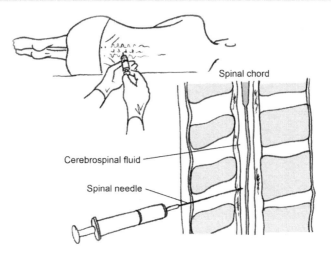

FIGURE 5.5 Lumbar puncture.

Postoperative considerations
- CSF is sent for analysis (biochemistry, bacteriology +/– cytology).
- Patient should remain flat for the next 4–6 hours.

Additional considerations
Contraindications:
- Raised intracranial pressure (if suspected, perform a CT head scan prior to the procedure).
- Known or suspected intracranial mass.
- Suspicion of a spinal cord or posterior fossa mass.
- Non-communicating hydrocephalus.
- Local infection near lumbar puncture site.
- Coagulopathy or patients on anticoagulation (e.g. heparin, warfarin, aspirin).
- Children with a tethered spinal cord.
- Patients with complete spinal block (relative).

CONSENT FORM
Name of procedure: Lumbar puncture (spinal tap)
Benefits:
  Diagnostic:
      Collection and analysis of cerebrospinal fluid (CSF) for infection (meningitis), blood (subarachnoid haemorrhage), abnormal protein (myeloma), and malignant cells
      Injection of contrast (myelogram)
      Measurement of opening pressure
  Therapeutic:
      Drainage of CSF
      Administration of intrathecal medication (e.g. chemotherapy and antibiotics)
      Preliminary step for the insertion of a spinal drain

Risks:
The overall risk of disabling or persistent neurological symptoms is estimated at 0.1%–0.5%.[1] Severe side-effects are rare[2] – brainstem herniation, infection, subdural haematoma.

General:
Headache (2%–40%), higher after diagnostic LP than epidural anaesthesia[3]
Bleeding into the subarachnoid or subdural space
Infection (spinal meningitis)

Specific:
Nerve root injury
Tonsillar herniation 1.2%[4]
Spinal epidural haematoma
Spinal epidural CSF collection
Epidermoid tumour
Intracranial subdural hygroma or haematoma

Procedure involves: General/regional/local anaesthesia

Key publications

Kuntz KM, Kokmen E, Stevens JC, *et al*. Post-lumbar puncture headaches: experience in 501 consecutive procedures. *Neurology*. 1992; **42**: 1884–7.[5]

- All adults who underwent an ambulatory lumbar puncture (LP) in a 1-year period.
- Patients completed a questionnaire detailing their headache experience on the day of and day 6 following the LP.
- Patients reporting headaches before the LP were more likely to report post-procedure LP headaches.
- Younger female patients with a lower body mass index have the highest risk of developing post-lumbar puncture headaches (PLPHA).
- CSF opening pressure, cells, protein, patient's position during LP, the duration of recumbency following LP, the amount of CSF removed at the time of LP, did not influence the occurrence of headache.

Evans RW, Armon C, Frohman EM, *et al*. Assessment: prevention of post-lumbar puncture headaches: report of the Therapeutics and Technology Assessment Subcommittee of the American Academy of Neurology. *Neurology*. 2000; **55**(7): 909–14.[6]

- Review of the literature demonstrated that the use of an atraumatic spinal needle in adult patient population reduces the frequency of post-lumbar puncture headaches. It affirmed that smaller needle size was associated with reduced frequency of PLPHA (level A recommendation). *Also see* ref. 7.

References

1 Wiesel J, Rose DN, Silver AL, *et al*. Lumbar puncture in asymptomatic late syphilis. an analysis of benefits and risks. *Arch Intern Med*. 1985; **145**: 465–8.
2 Fishman RA. *Cerebrospinal Fluid in Diseases of the Nervous System*. Philadelphia, PA: WB Saunders; 1992.
3 Digiovanni AJ, Dunbar BS. Epidural injections of autologous blood for post-lumbar puncture headache. *Anesth Analg*. 1970; **49**: 268–71.
4 Korein J, Cravioto H, Leicach M. Revaluation of lumbar puncture: a study of 129 patients with papilledema or intracranial hypertension. *Neurology*. 1959; **9**: 290–7.

5 Kuntz KM, Kokmen E, Stevens JC, *et al.* Post-lumbar puncture headaches: experience in 501 consecutive procedures. *Neurology.* 1992; **42**: 1884–7.

6 Evans RW, Armon C, Frohman EM, *et al.* Assessment: prevention of post-lumbar puncture headaches: report of the Therapeutics and Technology Assessment Subcommittee of the American Academy of Neurology. *Neurology.* 2000; **55**(7): 909–14.

7 Armon C, Evans RW. Addendum to assessment: prevention of post-lumbar puncture headaches: report of the Therapeutics and Technology Assessment Subcommittee of the American Academy of Neurology. *Neurology.* 2005; **65**(4): 510–12.

Otolaryngology

6.1 Myringotomy and grommets
Key points
A myringotomy is an incision in the tympanic membrane (eardrum or pars tensa), with or without insertion of a grommet (also known as a ventilation tube or tympanostomy tube), with the aim of ventilating the middle ear space. Common indications include otitis media with effusion ('glue ear') and recurrent acute suppurative otitis media.

Procedural considerations
- Up-to-date preoperative pure tone audiometry (within 3 months of procedure).
- Day-case procedure.
- General anaesthesia, or local anaesthesia (EMLA or Ametop in external auditory canal).[1] The latter is an option in some adults.
- Microsuction clearance of the external auditory canal in order to visualise and examine the entirety of the tympanic membrane. A myringotomy incision is made in the safe part of the tympanic membrane – usually the antero-inferior quadrant. Any glue or pus in the middle ear space is microsuctioned. If indicated a grommet is inserted through the myringotomy incision.

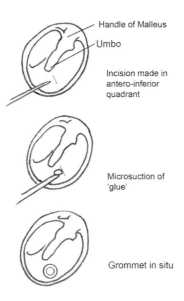

Handle of Malleus

Umbo

Incision made in antero-inferior quadrant

Microsuction of 'glue'

Grommet in situ

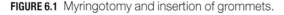

FIGURE 6.1 Myringotomy and insertion of grommets.

Postoperative considerations
- Dry ear precautions.
- Avoid diving (but shallow water swimming in fresh water is OK).
- Age-appropriate hearing test (pure tone audiometry and tympanometry) at 6 weeks' postop.

Additional considerations
Alternative/adjuvant treatments and outcomes:
- Watch and wait vs. hearing aids.
- 12 weeks of conservative management before active management.[2]
- Role of adjuvant adenoidectomy in improving eustachian tube dysfunction is still open to debate, although there is some evidence of benefit from the TARGET trial (trial of alternative regimens in glue ear treatment).[3]
- Hearing aids preferred to grommets in children with Down's syndrome and otitis media with effusion resulting in hearing loss (NICE guidelines).[4] The insertion of ventilation tubes is a less-favourable option for children with Down's syndrome as they are more susceptible to subsequent otorrhoea and there is a higher extrusion rate. In addition, insertion of ventilation tubes is made more difficult by the often small size of the external auditory canals. A number will also have a coexisting sensorineural hearing loss which must be identified.

CONSENT FORM
Name of procedure: EUA ears + myringotomies +/− insertion of grommets
Benefits:
> Improve symptoms (hearing, infections)

Risks:
> **General:**
>> Bleeding
>> Infection
> **Specific:**
>> Discharging ears
>> Residual/persistent perforation:
>>> Shah grommets: 1%–3%
>>> T-tubes: up to 50%
>> Repeat grommets

Procedure involves: General anaesthesia or local anaesthesia

Key publications
Nichani J, Camilleri AE, Broomfield S, *et al*. Optimizing local anaesthesia for grommet insertion: eutectic mixture of local anaesthetics versus Ametop: a randomized clinical trial. *Otol Neurotol*. 2008; **29**(5): 658–60.[1]
- Double-blind randomised controlled trial.
- 41 patients.
- Randomised to receive either EMLA (n=21), or Ametop (n=20).
- Primary outcome measure – level of pain experienced.
- Secondary outcome measure – overall procedural satisfaction.
- No statistically significant difference in pain or satisfaction scores between the two

groups, with the authors concluding that both topical anaesthetic agents provide good pain relief during grommet insertion.

- However, topical anaesthesia does not anaesthetise the medial surface of the tympanic membrane and the middle ear.

References
1 Nichani J, Camilleri AE, Broomfield S, *et al*. Optimizing local anaesthesia for grommet insertion: eutectic mixture of local anaesthetics versus Ametop: a randomized clinical trial. *Otol Neurotol*. 2008; **29**(5): 658–60.
2 Browning GG. Watchful waiting in childhood otitis media with effusion. *Clin Otolaryngol Allied Sci*. 2001; **26**(4): 263–4.
3 Medical Research Council Multicentre Otitis Media Study Group. Surgery for persistent otitis media with effusion: generalizability of results from the UK trial (TARGET). Trial of Alternative Regimens in Glue Ear Treatment. *Clin Otolaryngol Allied Sci*. 2001; **26**(5): 417–24.
4 National Institute for Health and Clinical Excellence. Surgical Management of Otitis Media with Effusion in Children: NICE guideline 60. London: NIHCE; 2008. http://guidance.nice.org.uk/CG60/NICEGuidance/doc/English (accessed 13 June 2010).

6.2 Nasal cautery
Key points
Nasal cautery is the use of chemical agents (usually silver nitrate), or electrocautery (usually monopolar diathermy) to seal bleeding vessels in Little's area (Kiesselbach's plexus) in order to treat or prevent epistaxis.

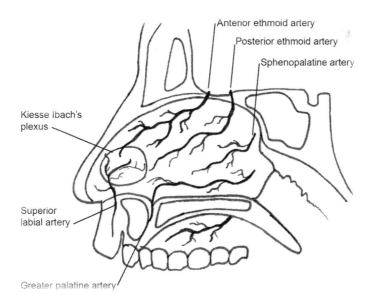

Anterior ethmoid artery
Posterior ethmoid artery
Sphenopalatine artery
Kiesse lbach's plexus
Superior labial artery
Greater palatine artery

FIGURE 6.2 Little's area – anterior nasal septal site of anastomosis (Kiesselbach's plexus) between the sphenopalatine, anterior ethmoidal, greater palatine and superior labial arteries.

Procedural considerations

- Outpatient department procedure under local anaesthetic spray containing 5% lignocaine and 0.5% phenylephrine (for silver nitrate cautery), or day-case procedure under general anaesthetic (diathermy).
- Perform anterior rhinoscopy with a Thudicum's speculum to visualise Little's area. The vessel responsible for bleeding will stand out from the mucosa as a prominent blood vessel.
- The prominent bleeding blood vessel, and its feeding vessels, are cauterised using the following technique:
  - first encircle the bleeding vessel itself (this cauterises the feeding vessels first)
  - then cauterise the prominent bleeding blood vessel itself.
- The silver nitrate stick will react with the mucosa and produce a grey eschar.
- If the bleeding site is not visible, it may be a posterior bleed.
- Cauterising both sides of the septum in the same sitting is contraindicated as there is a genuine risk of a causing a septal perforation. Therefore, an interval of at least 6 weeks is recommended before cauterising the contralateral side.

Postoperative considerations

- Application of Naseptin ointment for 10 days. (NB: contraindicated in patients with peanut allergies!)
- No nose picking!
- Avoidance of hot baths, hot showers, straining and heavy exercise.
- No nose blowing; sneeze through the mouth (rather than nose).
- Recommend a blood pressure check with the patient's GP, if necessary.
- Usual first aid measures apply in the case of a re-bleed (pinching fleshy part of the nose, head forwards, application of ice packs).[1]
- If ongoing bleeding, return to the emergency department for an ENT review +/– nasal packing.

Additional considerations

- Check full blood count and clotting (persistent, or recurrent epistaxis). In emergency situations, assess for evidence of haemorrhagic shock, and group and save, and/or cross-match blood.
- EUA nose and postnasal space using nasendoscope to exclude other causes (e.g. juvenile nasal angiofibromas in young males).
- Alternative treatments and outcomes:
  - Nasal packing, arterial angiogram and embolisation (radiological), surgical procedures including endoscopic sphenopalatine artery ligation, anterior ethmoidal artery ligation, maxillary artery ligation, external carotid artery ligation.[2]

CONSENT FORM
Name of procedure: EUA nose + nasal cautery
Benefits:
  Diagnosis
  Prevent nosebleeds (epistaxis)
Risks:
  General:
    Nosebleed
    Infection

Specific:
   Septal perforation
Procedure involves: Local anaesthetic spray (silver nitrate cautery) or general
   anaesthetic (monopolar diathermy)

Key publications

Fishman JM, Brooks A, Banfield G. Patient perceptions of appropriate first aid measures
in epistaxis management and the effect of brief interventions. *Rhinology.* 2009; **47**: 332.[1]
* Questionnaire-based study in the outpatient ENT department.
* 285 patients asked a multitude of questions relating to appropriate first aid measures
  in epistaxis and scored accordingly.
* 194 of the 285 participants (68%) thought incorrectly that the hard bony portion of
  the nose should be pinched in epistaxis.
* The study should assist in educating patients regarding correct epistaxis first aid
  management.

Moshaver A, Harris JR, Liu R, *et al.* Early operative intervention versus conventional
treatment in epistaxis: randomized prospective trial. *J Otolaryngol.* 2004; **33**(3): 185–8.[2]
* Prospective randomised trial.
* Intranasal endoscopic sphenopalatine artery ligation vs. conventional nasal packing
  in the treatment of recurrent epistaxis.
* Small sample size (n=19).
* Significant reduction in length of stay in hospital and overall cost in the surgical
  group compared with the conservative arm of the study.
* Surgery 89% effective in controlling epistaxis with minimal complication rate.
* The method of randomisation was not discussed and no reasons for withdrawals
  were provided, making it difficult to judge the internal validity of the study.
* Power calculations were not reported, and the sample size seems to have been
  relatively small. Thus, it was not possible to ascertain whether the results were due to
  the intervention or to chance.

References

1 Fishman JM, Brooks A, Banfield G. Patient perceptions of appropriate first aid measures in epistaxis management and the effect of brief interventions. *Rhinology.* 2009;
   47: 332.
2 Moshaver A, Harris JR, Liu R, *et al.* Early operative intervention versus conventional
   treatment in epistaxis: randomized prospective trial. *J Otolaryngol.* 2004; **33**(3): 185–8.

6.3 Drainage of a quinsy: needle aspiration
Key points
A quinsy is a peritonsillar abscess (a collection of pus in the peritonsillar space).

Procedural considerations
* Always consider the need for airway protection – especially if there is a large abscess.
* Emergency department procedure under local anaesthetic (xylocaine spray).
* Needle aspiration of a quinsy is performed with a large bore needle (from a

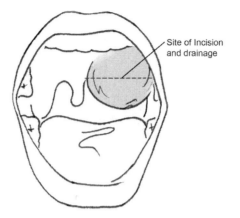

Site of Incision and drainage

FIGURE 6.3 The reliable clinical signs of a quinsy include asymmetrical tonsils, medialisation of the tonsil, deviation of the uvula to the contralateral side, associated trismus, peritonsillar oedema/cellulitis/pus/exudate.[1]

large cannula) on a 10 mL syringe, with the aid of a good headlight and a tongue depressor.[7]
- The needle is inserted into the most fluctuant area of the quinsy, the pus drained and sent for microscopy, culture and sensitivity.
- If a dry tap is obtained on the first pass, up to two further attempts should be made in neighbouring areas (in case of a loculated abscess).

Postoperative considerations
- Often requires inpatient admission following aspiration, or incision and drainage, for intravenous antibiotics, fluids, analgesia +/– intravenous steroids.[3]
- Can go home when eating and drinking, with resolution of symptoms and signs.[4]
- Two episodes of quinsy justifies an elective tonsillectomy. One episode of quinsy justifies a tonsillectomy on a background history of recurrent tonsillitis. Patient choice is important.

Additional considerations
Quinsies usually occur in younger age groups. A malignant lesion should be excluded in elderly patients (especially smokers).
   Alternative treatments and outcomes:
- Incision and drainage with a guarded blade. (NB: The internal carotid artery lies 2.5 cm posterolateral to the tonsillar bed.[5])
- 'Hot' (quinsy) tonsillectomy under general anaesthetic – if quinsy fails to resolve with medical management, if unable to aspirate/drain due to poor cooperation (e.g. young children), associated complications (e.g. parapharyngeal abscess).[5]

CONSENT FORM
Name of procedure: Aspiration or incision and drainage of a quinsy
Benefits:
      Relief of symptoms (pain, odynophagia, 'hot potato' voice)
Risks:
  General:
      Bleeding
  Specific:
      Aspiration of pus
      Recurrence: 10%–15%[5]
Procedure involves: Local anaesthetic spray

Key publications

Kilty SJ, Gaboury I. Clinical predictors of peritonsillar abscess in adults. *J Otolaryngol Head Neck Surg.* 2008; **37**(2): 165–0.[1]
- Observational study.
- Review of 130 patients with either a peritonsillar abscess or simple tonsillitis (age range 16–91).
- 50 patients diagnosed with a peritonsillar abscess; 80 with tonsillitis.
- Clinical signs significantly associated with peritonsillar abscess (rather than tonsillitis) included trismus ($p<0.001$), uvular deviation ($p<0.001$), and inferior displacement of the superior pole of the tonsil ($p<0.001$) on the affected side. Pain duration was not a significant discriminative factor.

Ozbek C, Aygenc E, Tuna EU, *et al.* Use of steroids in the treatment of peritonsillar abscess. *J Laryngol Otol.* 2004; **118**(6): 439–42.[3]
- Doubled-blind prospective randomised study.
- 62 patients hospitalised after aspiration of quinsy.
- One arm received intravenous antibiotic therapy and a single dose placebo (n=28).
- The other group received a single, high dose of steroid in addition to intravenous antibiotic (n=34).
- Outcomes included length of stay in hospital, throat pain, fever, trismus, dysphagia.
- There was a statistically significant difference between the two groups ($p<0.01$), indicating that single use of high dose steroid as an adjunct to antibiotic therapy is more effective than use of antibiotics alone.

Al Yaghchi C, Cruise A, Kapoor K, *et al.* Out-patient management of patients with a peritonsillar abscess. *Clin Otolaryngol.* 2008; **33**(1): 52–5.[4]
- Observational study.
- 44 patients treated with quinsy and managed in the outpatient setting.
- 41 were happy to have been treated as outpatients and not admitted to hospital (93%).
- The authors conclude that patients with a peritonsillar abscess can be managed successfully as outpatients with a high degree of patient satisfaction.
- However, most UK ENT departments will still admit patients with a peritonsillar abscess.

Johnson RF, Stewart MG, Wright CC. An evidence-based review of the treatment of peritonsillar abscess. *Otolaryngol Head Neck Surg.* 2003; **128**(3): 332–43.[5]

- Systematic review.
- 42 articles in the literature analysed.
- Five level I studies on surgical technique identified, which indicated that needle aspiration, incision and drainage, and quinsy ('hot') tonsillectomy are all equally effective for the initial management of peritonsillar abscess.
- Overall recurrence rate of peritonsillar abscess is 10%–15%.

References

1 Kilty SJ, Gaboury I. Clinical predictors of peritonsillar abscess in adults. *J Otolaryngol Head Neck Surg.* 2008; **37**(2): 165–8.
2 Leong SC. Demystifying the technique of aspirating a quinsy. *Clin Otolaryngol.* 2007; **32**(2): 140–1.
3 Ozbek C, Aygenc E, Tuna EU, *et al.* Use of steroids in the treatment of peritonsillar abscess. *J Laryngol Otol.* 2004; **118**(6): 439–42.
4 Al Yaghchi C, Cruise A, Kapoor K, *et al.* Out-patient management of patients with a peritonsillar abscess. *Clin Otolaryngol.* 2008; **33**(1): 52–5.
5 Johnson RF, Stewart MG, Wright CC. An evidence-based review of the treatment of peritonsillar abscess. *Otolaryngol Head Neck Surg.* 2003; **128**(3): 332–43.

6.4 Adenotonsillectomy

Key points

The palatine tonsils ('tonsils') and pharyngeal tonsils ('adenoids') are aggregate collections of lymphoid tissue that together form part of Waldeyer's ring and may become important sites of pathological disease. Tonsillectomy is surgical excision of the palatine tonsils, while adenoidectomy is excision of the pharyngeal tonsils (adenoids).

Procedural considerations

- Preoperative assessment – exclude family history of bleeding diathesis, check full blood count, clotting, sickle cell status if indicated.
- Day case (kept for at least 6 hours post-recovery due to a risk of delayed primary or reactionary haemorrhage), or overnight stay if performed late in the day.

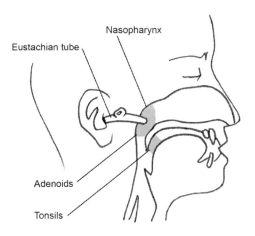

FIGURE 6.4 Adenoids and tonsils.

- General anaesthetic.
- The mouth is held open through the use of a Boyle–Davis mouth gag and Draffin rods. Adenoids may be curetted or removed by suction diathermy. Removal of tonsils is usually performed by one of a combination of techniques including cold steel and ties, bipolar diathermy and/or Coblation.

Postoperative considerations
- Return to theatre if primary haemorrhage.
- Encourage eating and drinking, with use of regular analgesia.
- Two weeks off school/work.
- Return to emergency department if any late bleeding.

Additional considerations
Common indications for tonsillectomy:
- Recurrent acute tonsillitis.
- History of peritonsillar abscess.
- Obstructive sleep apnoea/snoring.
- For diagnosis (e.g. squamous cell carcinoma, lymphoma).

Common indications for adenoidectomy:
- To improve symptoms of adenoidal hypertrophy and adenoiditis.
- Obstructive sleep apnoea and snoring.
- To improve eustachian tube function.
- For diagnostic purposes.

CONSENT FORM
Name of procedure: Tonsillectomy and/or adenoidectomy
Benefits:
 Improve symptoms (e.g. tonsillitis, breathing, snoring)
 +/– diagnosis[1]
Risks:
 General:
  Bleeding:
   Primary haemorrhage: 0.6%[2]
   Secondary haemorrhage: 3%[2]
  Infection
 Specific:
  Tooth damage
  Rhinolalia aperta (hypernasal speech following adenoidectomy)
  Lymphoid regrowth (adenoids)
Procedure involves: General anaesthetic

Key publications
Burton MJ, Glasziou PP. Tonsillectomy or adeno-tonsillectomy versus non-surgical treatment for chronic/recurrent acute tonsillitis. Cochrane Database Syst Rev. 2009; 1: CD001802.[1]
- Systematic review and meta-analysis.

- Includes five studies: four undertaken in children (719 participants) and one in adults (70 participants).
- Adeno-/tonsillectomy is effective in reducing the number of episodes of sore throat and days with sore throats in children, the gain being more marked in those most severely affected.

References
1 Burton MJ, Glasziou PP. Tonsillectomy or adeno-tonsillectomy versus non-surgical treatment for chronic/recurrent acute tonsillitis. Cochrane Database Syst Rev. 2009; 1: CD001802.
2 The Royal College of Surgeons of England. *National Prospective Tonsillectomy Audit.* London: RCSE; 2005. Available at: www.rcseng.ac.uk/rcseng/content/publications/docs/national_prospective.html

6.5 Reduction of simple nasal fractures
Key points
A manipulation of a nasal fracture under anaesthetic is required following injury to improve cosmesis and/or nasal obstruction. It requires closed reduction and immobilisation.

Procedural considerations
- Exclude a septal haematoma and cerebrospinal fluid leak, both of which can complicate a nasal fracture, in addition to signs of a blowout fracture of the orbit – crepitus, numbness in distribution of infraorbital nerves, ophthalmoplegia (painful/restricted eye movements, diplopia).
- Signs of a fractured nose include one or more of the following: brisk epistaxis at time of injury, periorbital ecchymosis, oedema, nasal tenderness, new nasal deformity, and new nasal obstruction.
- Review the patient in the ENT clinic approximately 7 days following injury when the swelling has subsided (unless presenting immediately after injury in which case a manipulation may be performed immediately).

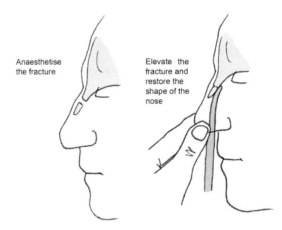

Anaesthetise the fracture

Elevate the fracture and restore the shape of the nose

FIGURE 6.5 Manipulation of simple nasal fracture.

- Check for a history of nasal trauma and previous nasal surgery (reduces chances of success of procedure).
- Ensure manipulation under anaesthetic (MUA) takes place within 3 weeks following injury so that the fracture line remains 'soft'.
- Day-case procedure under general anaesthetic, or can be performed under local anaesthetic in the outpatient department.[1]
- The fracture is reduced manually with the aid of Walsham's forceps, or a Hill's elevator. Steristrips are placed over the dorsum of the nose to reduce swelling.
- The nose is immobilised with plaster of Paris, or an external nasal (Denver) splint.

Postoperative considerations
- If manipulation of the nose causes bleeding, which is uncommon, the nose can be packed temporarily and the patient observed for a few hours.
- Leave plaster, or splint, on for 1 week. Then advise the patient to wear it at night only for up to a further 6 weeks to prevent redisplacement.
- Avoid contact sports for 6 weeks to prevent redisplacement.

Additional considerations
Alternative treatments and outcomes:
- Local anaesthetic nerve blocks, or general anaesthetic (MUA).
- Formal septorhinoplasty (open reduction) with osteotomies if delay in presentation, or if malunion persists despite MUA and closed reduction.

CONSENT FORM
Name of procedure: Manipulation under anaesthesia of nasal fracture
Benefits:
    Cosmesis
    Improve nasal blockage
Risks:
  General:
    Bruising and swelling
  Specific:
    Plaster/splint postop
    Nosebleed
    Persistent deformity/unsuccessful attempt
    Formal septoplasty/rhinoplasty/septorhinoplasty if unsuccessful (3.2% if first MUA under GA, 17.2% if first MUA under LA[3])
Procedure involves: Local anaesthetic nerve blocks, or general anaesthetic

---

Key publications
Chadha NK, Repanos C, Carswell AJ. Local anaesthesia for manipulation of nasal fractures: systematic review. *J Laryngol Otol.* 2009; **123**(8): 830–6.[1]
- Systematic review and meta-analysis.
- Included randomised controlled trials comparing general anaesthesia with local anaesthesia, or comparing different local anaesthetic techniques.
- No significant differences were found between local and general anaesthesia with respect to cosmesis, pain or nasal patency.

- The least painful local anaesthetic method was topical tetracaine gel applied to the nasal dorsum together with topical intranasal cocaine solution.
- Minimal adverse events were reported with the use of local anaesthesia.
- The authors conclude that local anaesthesia appears to be a safe and effective alternative to general anaesthesia for analgesia during nasal fracture manipulation, with no evidence of inferior outcomes.

References

1 Chadha NK, Repanos C, Carswell AJ. Local anaesthesia for manipulation of nasal fractures: systematic review. *J Laryngol Otol.* 2009; **123**(8): 830–6.
2 Panesar J, Panagamuwa C, Pitchard M, *et al.* How to block and tackle a fractured nose using local anaesthetic. *CME Bull Otorhinolaryngol Head Neck Surg.* 2004; **8**(2): 65–7.
3 Courtney MJ, Rajapakse Y, Duncan G, *et al.* Nasal fracture manipulation: a comparative study of general and local anaesthesia techniques. *Clin Otolaryngol Allied Sci.* 2003; **28**(5): 472–5.

Paediatric surgery

7.1 Circumcision
Key points
Circumcision is excision of the foreskin. It is the commonest paediatric surgical procedure and is usually performed for cultural or religious reasons. The medical indications include pathological phimosis, recurrent balanitis and congenital urogenital malformations that predispose to urinary tract infection. Pathological phimosis is the pathological narrowing of the preputial orifice resulting in inability to retract the prepuce over the glans penis. This is unusual under 5 years of age.[1] It must be differentiated from physiological phimosis due to preputial adhesions, which results in non-retractable foreskin often up to the age of 3 years.[1]

Procedural considerations
- Day-case procedure.
- General anaesthesia with or without penile block.
- Plastibell: adhesions between the prepuce and glans are freed, the prepuce is fully retracted, and the Plastibell is placed over the glans and the prepuce drawn up over it. A tight suture is placed around the foreskin over the groove in the device. The foreskin necroses off within 3–7 days.
- Freehand: the phimosis is dilated and adhesions between prepuce and glans broken down. A circular incision is made in the inner prepuce, just proximal to the coronal groove and a second incision is made on the outer foreskin. The skin between both incisions is excised, haemostasis achieved and the wound is closed.

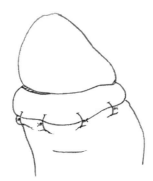

FIGURE 7.1 Circumcision.

Postoperative considerations
- Regular topical antibiotic (chloramphenicol 1%) to glans to prevent sticking to underclothes.
- Return to school in 7–10 days.

Additional considerations
Alternative treatments:
- Dorsal slit – dorsal foreskin incision that exposes the glans. Unsatisfactory cosmesis.
- Topical steroid therapy – 65.8%–95% success rate reported. Proposed mechanisms of action: skin thinning, reduced production of inflammatory mediators, lubricant effect.[2]
- GMC guidance states that permission from both parents should be obtained 'whenever possible' when obtaining consent for non-medical circumcision of boys.[3] A single centre retrospective study found written consent from both parents was obtained in only 6.4% of cases.[4] This was attributed partly to ignorance of the rules.

CONSENT FORM
Name of procedure: Circumcision
Benefits:
  Treatment of phimosis/recurrent balanitis
  Relieve symptoms
  Prevent disease progression
Risks:
  Bleeding: 1%[6]
  Infection
  Excision of inadequate or excess foreskin
  Meatal ulcer
  Meatal stenosis – which may require further surgery in the future: 3%–11%[5]
  Urethral damage/fistula
  Injury to glans
Procedure involves: General anaesthesia and/or regional anaesthesia

---

Key publications
Cathcart P, Nuttall M, van der Meulen J, *et al.* Trends in paediatric circumcision and its complications in England between 1997 and 2003. *Br J Surg.* 2006; **93**(7): 885–90.[6]
- Retrospective cohort study.
- 75 868 boys under the age of 15 included in the study.
- Data extracted from the Hospital Episode Statistics database of admission to NHS hospitals in England.
- There was a 20% fall in circumcision rate from 1997 to 2003. In 2003 it was 2.1 per 1000 boys.
- Indications for circumcision: 90% phimosis, 8% balanitis, 2% other.
- 1.2% of boys experienced complications.
- The study excluded boys who had additional operative procedures at time of circumcision.
- Only complications requiring prolonged hospital stay or readmission included therefore some minor complications not included in the study.

Esposito C, Centonze A, Alicchio F, *et al*. Topical steroid application versus circumcision in pediatric patients with phimosis: a prospective randomized placebo-controlled clinical trial. *World J Urol*. 2008; **26**(2): 187–90.[2]

- Prospective study.
- 240 boys.
- Randomised to placebo cream or steroid cream (monometasone furoate 0.1%) twice a day for 4 weeks.
- At median follow up of 20 months, therapeutic success was obtained in 65.8% of cases in the steroid-cream-treated group and 16.6% of the placebo-treated group (statistically significant difference).
- No complications from treatment reported.

References
1 The Royal College of Surgeons of England, *et al*. *Male circumcision: guidance for healthcare practitioners*. Statement from the British Association of Paediatric Surgeons, the Royal College of Nursing, the Royal College of Paediatrics and Child Health, The Royal College of Surgeons of England and the Royal College of Anaesthetists. London: Royal College of Surgeons of England; May 2000. Available at: www.rcseng.ac.uk/publications/docs/male_circumcision.html

2 Esposito C, Centonze A, Alicchio F, *et al*. Topical steroid application versus circumcision in pediatric patients with phimosis: a prospective randomized placebo-controlled clinical trial. *World J Urol*. 2008; **26**(2): 187–90.

3 General Medical Council. *Guidance for doctors who are asked to circumcise male children*. London: GMC; 1997.

4 Robinson R, Makin E, Wheeler R. Consent for non-therapeutic male circumcision on religious grounds. *Ann R Coll Surg Engl*. 2009; **91**(2): 152–4.

5 Van Howe RS. Incidence of meatal stenosis following neonatal circumcision in a primary care setting. *Clin Pediatr (Phila)*. 2006; **45**(1): 49–54.

6 Cathcart P, Nuttall M, van der Meulen J, *et al*. Trends in paediatric circumcision and its complications in England between 1997 and 2003. *Br J Surg*. 2006; **93**(7): 885–90.

7.2 Operative reduction of intussusception
Key points
Intussusception is invagination of a segment of intestine (intussusceptum) into the lumen of adjacent more distal bowel (intussuscipiens). This results in venous congestion and bowel wall oedema. It is ileo-colic in approximately 80% of cases and ileo-ilial in approximately 15%. It occurs mostly between 2 months and 2 years of age, with the highest incidence at 4–10 months and is the commonest cause of bowel obstruction in this age group. Over 90% cases are idiopathic. There is a suggested causal link with viral respiratory and enteric infections. Symptoms include vomiting, colicky pain and bloody stools but they occur together in less than a quarter of patients.[1]

Procedural considerations
- Preoperative fluid resuscitation, FBC, U&Es, blood group and antibody screen.
- Diagnosis is usually made on ultrasound examination (sensitivity of 98% and specificity of 100%).
- Reduction by enema is usually attempted before surgical reduction unless contraindicated.
- Indications for surgery: initial evidence of perforation or peritonism, failed air

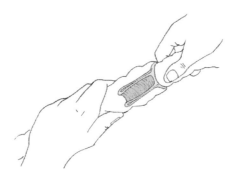

FIGURE 7.2 Reduction of intussusception.

enema reduction, perforation during enema reduction, third presentation or presentation outside of usual age range.
- Operative reduction is performed in 10%–28% of cases.[2,3]
- General anaesthesia.
- Open: a right transverse muscle cutting incision is made at the umbilical level. Intussusception is identified and reduced by gentle pushing on the distal bowel. The bowel is inspected for necrosis, perforation and pathological lead point. Resection and anastomosis are performed as required. Appendicectomy is usually also performed.
- Laparoscopic ports: 5 mm umbilical port for laparoscope, and two 3 mm or 5 mm working ports, one in left lower quadrant, other in left upper quadrant. Intussusception is identified. Reduction is achieved with atraumatic graspers by gently placing pressure distal to the intussusceptum in a squeezing fashion and gentle traction on bowel proximal to the intussusception followed by inspection for necrosis. If necessary, resection is performed via a small periumbilical incision or converted to an open procedure. Laparoscopy is safe if there are no initial signs of perforation, peritonitis and the patient is haemodynamically stable. Conversion to open occurs in 12.5%–50%.[4]
- Bowel resection is required in 23%–37% of cases.[5]

Postoperative considerations
- IV fluids.
- NG decompression.
- Start PO fluids at 24–48 hours postop.
- Antibiotics if required.
- Length of stay 3–6 days postop. Longer after open operation than laparoscopic.[2]

Additional considerations
- Air enema reduction usually attempted prior to surgical reduction. Successful in 75%–90% of cases.[6] Failure is more likely if symptoms have been present more than 24 hours or if there is absent colour flow seen on Doppler examination. Risk of perforation is <1%[6] and recurrence 5.4% to 15.4%.[6]
- Without treatment, advancing intussusception and increasing bowel oedema result in progression to necrosis of the bowel wall, perforation and death.[3]
- Spontaneous reduction without treatment is rare (2%).[3]

CONSENT FORM

Name of procedure: Laparotomy for reduction of intussusception +/– bowel resection +/– appendicectomy OR laparoscopic reduction of intussusception +/– conversion to open operation +/– bowel resection +/– appendicectomy

Benefits:
    Treat intussusception
    Prevent disease progression

Risks:
    Bleeding
    Infection – wound, abdominal abscess, sepsis, urinary tract, respiratory tract
    Perforation
    Recurrence of intussusception: 1%–6%[1,2]
    Anastomotic leak: 4%,[4] stricture: <1%[1,2]
    Prolonged ileus
    Bowel obstruction: 1%[1]
    Mortality: <1%[7]
    Scar

Procedure involves: General anaesthesia
Additional procedures: Blood transfusion

Key publications

Bailey KA, Wales PW, Gerstle JT. Laparoscopic versus open reduction of intussusception in children: a single-institution comparative experience. *J Pediatr Surg.* 2007; **42**(5): 845–8.[4]

- Retrospective review.
- 41 patients who underwent surgical treatment for intussusception at the Hospital for Sick Children in Toronto from January 2002 to February 2006.
- Age range 4–135 months.
- Use of laparoscopic (18) or open (23) approach was based surgeon's preference.
- Operative time not statistically different between laparoscopic and open groups.
- 28% of laparoscopic group patients converted to open.
- Length of stay statistically shorter in laparoscopic group (4.8 +/– 3.5 vs. 9.1+/– 7.5 days).
- Times to first feed and full feed significantly shorter in laparoscopic group.
- Complication rate not statistically different (22% laparoscopic group, 26% open group).

References

1 Kaiser AD, Applegate KE, Ladd AP. Current success in the treatment of intussusception in children. *Surgery.* 2007; **142**(4): 469–75.
2 Kia KF, Mony VK, Drongowski RA, *et al.* Laparoscopic vs. open surgical approach for intussusception requiring operative intervention. *J Pediatr Surg.* 2005; **40**(1): 281–4.
3 Lehnert T, Sorge I, Till H, *et al.* Intussusception in children: clinical presentation, diagnosis and management. *Int J Colorectal Dis.* 2009; **24**(10): 1187–92. Epub 2009 May 6.
4 Bailey KA, Wales PW, Gerstle JT. Laparoscopic versus open reduction of intussusception in children: a single-institution comparative experience. *J Pediatr Surg.* 2007; **42**(5): 845–8.

5 Somme S, To T, Langer JC. Factors determining the need for operative reduction in children with intussusception: a population-based study. *J Pediatr Surg*. 2006; **41**(5): 1014–9.

6 Daneman A, Navarro O. Intussusception Part 2: an update on the evolution of management. *Pediatr Radiol*. 2004; **34**(2): 97–108.

7 Stringer MD, Pablot SM, Brereton RJ. Paediatric intussusception. *Br J Surg*. 1992; **79**(9): 867–76.

7.3 Inguinal and umbilical hernia repair
Key points
Inguinal herniae – inguinal hernia repair is the commonest operation performed by paediatric surgeons.[1] They are more common in boys and usually on the right due to later testicular descent.[2] As the testis passes through the internal ring it brings a diverticulum of peritoneum (processus vaginalis) with it. The layers of the processus vaginalis usually fuse obliterating the entrance to the inguinal canal from the peritoneal cavity. Failure of this fusion results in an inguinal hernia. At presentation 75%–95% are unilateral.[1] In children who have an open repair the incidence of metachronous contralateral inguinal hernia is 7.2%.[1] There is debate regarding contralateral groin exploration and the use of laparoscopic repair.

Umbilical herniae – these are the commonest hernia in children and more common in girls. There is a defect in the umbilical ring due to failure of complete obliteration at the site where the foetal umbilical vessels enter the abdomen during gestation. The hernial sac protrudes through this defect. There is incomplete closure of the umbilical ring at birth in 20% of full-term neonates – 80% of umbilical herniae decrease in size and close spontaneously by 4–5 years of age.

Procedural considerations
- Day case.
- General/local anaesthesia.
- Inguinal hernia
  - Open: transverse incision is made in the inguinal skin crease. The superficial cord coverings are divided and the cremasteric muscle is identified over the cord. This is opened by blunt dissection to expose the hernial sac. The sac is lifted and the spermatic vessels and vas are dissected free from the cord. The sac is opened and any contents reduced. It is then twisted and transfixed. Closure in layers.

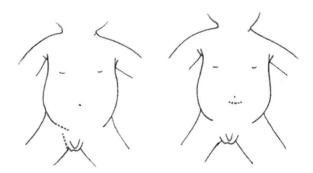

FIGURE 7.3 Incisions for hernia repair.

- Laparoscopic: camera is positioned above the umbilicus (5 mm port) and two instruments (3 mm) in right and left flanks without ports. Purse string suture is placed around the inner ring.
- Umbilical hernia
  - Curved incision is made in the crease below the umbilicus. Dissection is performed to the abdominal wall fascial layer and the plane around the base of hernia sac. Skin is dissected off the sac and the defect is closed. Skin margins are trimmed if required.

Postoperative considerations
- Resume oral intake on waking.
- Mild analgesia for 48 hours.
- Bath on third postoperative day.
- Return to normal activity 2.5 days.[3] No contact sports 10 days.
- Thickening or bruising of scrotum resolves in 1–2 weeks.
- Umbilical herniae: pledget and dressing swab placed in umbilicus to prevent haematoma formation.

Additional considerations
Inguinal herniae
- High risk of incarceration: overall rate in children 9%–20%. In infants it is up to 34%.[2]
- Incarceration leads to obstruction, strangulation and increased postoperative complications.[2]
- Complication rates higher in emergency repairs.
- Controversy over contralateral exploration: avoiding a second operation and reducing operative risks.[1] 14 contralateral explorations are required to prevent one metachronous hernia.[1]

Umbilical herniae
- Rupture or incarceration is exceptionally rare.
- Defects >1.5 cm rarely close spontaneously.

CONSENT FORM
Name of procedure: Inguinal hernia repair OR umbilical hernia repair
Benefits:
    Treat hernia
    Prevent complications of hernia (obstruction/strangulation)
Risks:
  General:
    Pain
    Scar
    Bleeding
    Wound infection: 1%–4%[4]
    Damage to intestine
  Specific:
  For inguinal hernia repair:
    Scrotal haematoma/postoperative hydrocoele
    Recurrent inguinal hernia: 0.9%–1.2%[5,6]

Iatrogenic cryptorchidism – testis may come to lie higher in the scrotum: <1%[5]

Injury to spermatic vessels leading to testicular atrophy: 0.2%–1.1%[2]

Injury to bladder: 0.3%[5]

Injury to vas deferens: 0.2%[5]

Injury to nerves

For umbilical hernia repair:

Seroma/haematoma formation

Recurrence (up to 3% if risk factors such as long-term ambulatory peritoneal dialysis, VP shunts, connective tissue disorder are present)[2]

Procedure involves: General anaesthesia and local anaesthesia

Additional procedures: Bowel resection (if operation is for an incarcerated hernia)

Key publications

Ron O, Eaton S, Pierro A. The systematic review of the risk of developing a metachronous contralateral inguinal hernia in children. *Br J Surg.* 2007; **94**(7): 804–11.[1]

- Systematic review.
- Inclusions – studies in which children underwent open repair of a unilateral inguinal hernia without contralateral exploration and were followed up for metachronous contralateral inguinal hernia.
- 49 papers analysed with data on 22 846 children.
- Incidence of metachronous contralateral inguinal hernia was 7.2% overall.
- Significantly higher risk of developing a metachronous contralateral inguinal hernia in children with a left-sided (10.2%) than those with a right-sided hernia (6.3%).
- Overall 14 contralateral explorations are required to prevent one metachronous hernia.
- Most metachronous contralateral inguinal hernias occur in the first 5 years after unilateral inguinal hernia repair.

Audry G, Johanet S, Achrafi H, *et al.* The risk of wound infection after inguinal incision in pediatric outpatient surgery. *Eur J Pediatr Surg.* 1994; **4**(2): 87–89.[4]

- Retrospective study.
- 2243 patients (1816 outpatients, 427 outpatients) undergoing an operation requiring an inguinal incision over 5.2 years.
- Wound infections in outpatients 18/1816 (0.1%), in inpatients 17/427 (4%).

References

1 Ron O, Eaton S, Pierro A. Systematic review of the risk of developing a metachronous contralateral inguinal hernia in children. *Br J Surg.* 2007; **94**(7): 804–11.

2 Meier AH, Ricketts RR. Surgical complications of inguinal and abdominal wall hernias. *Semin Pediatr Surg.* 2003; **12**(2): 89.

3 Koivusalo AI, Korpela R, Wirtavuori K, *et al.* A single-blinded, randomized comparison of laparoscopic versus open hernia repair in children. *Pediatrics.* 2009; **123**(1): 332–7.

4 Audry G, Johanet S, Achrafi H, *et al.* The risk of wound infection after inguinal incision in pediatric outpatient surgery. *Eur J Pediatr Surg.* 1994; **4**(2): 87–89.

5 Tiryaki T, Baskin D, Bulut M. Operative complications of hernia repair in childhood. *Pediatr Surg Int.* 1998 Mar; **13**(2–3): 160–1.

6 Ein SH, Njere I, Ein A. Six thousand three hundred sixty-one pediatric inguinal hernias: a 35-year review. *J Pediatr Surg.* 2006 May; **41**(5): 980–6.

7.4 Pyloromyotomy

Key points

Infantile hypertrophic pyloric stenosis is hypertrophy of the pyloric sphincter, causing non-bilious projectile vomiting that usually begins at 3–4 weeks of age. The infant is constantly hungry and there are visible gastric contractions and a palpable olive-shaped pyloric 'tumour' in the right upper quadrant. There is hyperchloraemic alkalosis and ultrasound is often used to confirm the diagnosis (pyloric muscle thickness >3 mm and pyloric canal length >17 mm). It is the commonest surgical cause of non-bilious vomiting in infants with an incidence of approximately 2–3/1000 live births in Caucasians. There is a male preponderance (4:1), often affecting first-born males, and a strong familial pattern of inheritance.

Procedural considerations

- NG tube to decompress stomach.
- Monitor U&Es and blood gases and correct dehydration and acid-base imbalance (may take up to 48–72 hr).
- General anaesthesia.
- Open
  - Transverse incision is made in right upper quadrant or curvilinear incision in the superior umbilical fold. Pyloric 'tumour' is identified by palpation and delivered out of the wound. Serosal incision is made along the length of the pyloric mass. Blunt instrument, e.g. handle of a scalpel is inserted into the hypertrophied muscle down to the submucosa. The muscle is split with a twisting action till the mucosa bulges out. Air is introduced into the stomach via the NG tube and milked into the duodenum to detect mucosal perforation.
- Laparoscopic
  - Camera port positioned at umbilicus and two instruments (3 mm) in the right and left upper quadrants. Duodenum is fixed with an atraumatic grasper and an incision is made along the length of the pylorus. A spreader is used to complete the myotomy till the mucosa bulges.

Postoperative considerations

- Continue IV fluids until feeding.
- Time to achieve full feeds is 18–24 hours postop (significantly shorter after laparoscopic compared with open procedure).[1]
- Length of stay is 33–44 hours postop (significantly shorter after laparoscopic compared with open).[1]

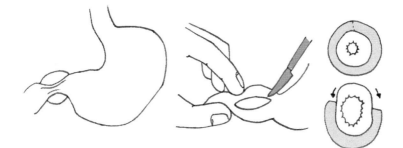

FIGURE 7.4 Pyloromyotomy.

Additional considerations
- Without any form of treatment, mortality rate approaches 100%.
- Intravenous atropine therapy is a possible alternative treatment. The treatment is long and there is uncertainty over the results. One study of 52 patients had an 87% success rate, however median hospital stay was 13 days and oral atropine medication had to be continued post discharge.[2]

CONSENT FORM

Name of procedure: Open pyloromyotomy OR laparoscopic pyloromyotomy +/– conversion to open

Benefits:
Treatment of pyloric stenosis

Risks:

General:
Bleeding
Wound infection: 3%–6%[1,3]
Adverse scarring
Pain

Specific:
Persistent postoperative vomiting (requiring further investigation): 4%[1]
Mucosal perforation: 2%[1]
Incomplete pyloromyotomy: 1%[3]

Procedure involves: General and local anaesthesia

Key publications
Hall NJ, Pacilli M, Eaton S, *et al*. Recovery after open versus laparoscopic pyloromyotomy for pyloric stenosis: a double-blind multicentre randomised controlled trial. *Lancet*. 2009; **373**: 390–8.[1]
- Randomised controlled trial.
- Double-blind, multicentre international trial (six tertiary paediatric surgical centres).
- 180 infants randomly assigned to open or laparoscopic pyloromyotomy.
- After laparoscopic pyloromyotomy, infants achieved full enteral feed more quickly than those undergoing open pyloromyotomy (18.5 hours vs. 23.9 hours, p=0.002).
- Postoperative length of stay was also shorter after laparoscopic pyloromyotomy than after open pyloromyotomy (33.6 hours vs. 43.8 hours, p=0.027).
- Postoperative vomiting, and intraoperative and postoperative complications, were similar between the two groups.
- Both open and laparoscopic pyloromyotomy were deemed safe procedures for the management of pyloric stenosis.
- However, laparoscopy has advantages over open pyloromyotomy and the authors of this study recommend its use in centres with suitable laparoscopic experience.

References
1 Hall NJ, Pacilli M, Eaton S, *et al*. Recovery after open versus laparoscopic pyloromyotomy for pyloric stenosis: a double-blind multicentre randomised controlled trial. *Lancet*. 2009; **373**: 390–8.
2 Kawahara H, Takama Y, Yoshida H, *et al*. Medical treatment of infantile hypertrophic

pyloric stenosis: should we always slice the 'olive'? *J Pediatr Surg.* 2005; **40**(12): 1848–51.

3 Allan C. Determinants of good outcome in pyloric stenosis. *J Paediatr Child Health.* 2006; **42**(3): 86–8.

7.5 EUA of rectum and manual evacuation
Key points
Constipation accounts for an estimated 3%–10% of visits to healthcare professionals by children.[1] Constipation is 'a delay or difficulty in defaecation, present for two or more weeks, sufficient to cause significant distress to the patient.'[2] A faecal mass or faecaloma may develop in the rectum after a few weeks of inefficient bowel action. This may result in continuous soiling from passage of small portions of the faecaloma through a partially open anus or liquid faeces flowing around the faecaloma. The faecaloma may be palpable abdominally. Management of paediatric faecal impaction entails emptying the constipated bowel and keeping it empty.[1]

Procedural considerations
* General anaesthetic.
* Digital examination of the rectum is performed to assess rectal tone and confirm presence of rectal distension or impaction.[2]
* The faecaloma is removed in small pieces.
* An anal dilatation or open rectal biopsy may also be performed – consent needs to be obtained for these procedures (not covered here).

Postoperative considerations
* After relief of impaction regular passage of soft stool should be maintained with the ongoing use of stool softeners or bulking agents and stimulants.[3]

Additional considerations
* There are no randomised controlled studies comparing methods of disimpaction.[2]
* Enemas (mineral oil, normal saline or hypertonic phosphate) can be used to disimpact. Risks include abdominal cramping, electrolyte imbalance and mechanical trauma.[2]

CONSENT FORM
Name of procedure: Rectal examination under anaesthetic and manual evacuation of rectum

Benefits:
      Evacuation of impacted faeces
      Relief of symptoms

Risks:
      Incomplete evacuation
      Anal stretch (this may be therapeutic if there is an associated anal fissure)
      Structural injury to the anal sphincter, which may contribute to sphincter weakness[4]

Procedure involves: General anaesthesia

Key publications

Gattuso JM, Kamm MA, Halligan SM, *et al*. The anal sphincter in idiopathic megarectum: effects of manual disimpaction under general anesthetic. *Dis Colon Rectum*. 1996; **39**(4): 435–9.[4]

- Retrospective cohort study.
- 17 adult patients with history of faecal impactions studied by anal endosonography and manometry when not impacted.
- 9 of 14 patients who had previously been manually disimpacted under general anaesthetic had disruption of one or both anal sphincter muscles on endosonography.
- Low anal resting pressure, indicative of internal sphincter dysfunction, was found in a substantial proportion of patients with either an endosonographically intact or disrupted internal anal sphincter.

References

1 Guest JF, Clegg JP. Modelling the costs and consequences of treating paediatric faecal impaction in Australia. *Curr Med Res Opin*. 2006; **22**(1): 107–19.
2 Biggs WS, Dery WH. Evaluation and treatment of constipation in infants and children. *Am Fam Physician*. 2006; **73**(3): 469–77.
3 Griffin SJ, Parkinson EJ, Malone PS. Bowel management for paediatric patients with faecal incontinence. *J Pediatr Urol*. 2008; **4**(5): 387–92.
4 Gattuso JM, Kamm MA, Halligan SM, *et al*. The anal sphincter in idiopathic megarectum: effects of manual disimpaction under general anesthetic. *Dis Colon Rectum*. 1996; **39**(4): 435–9.

7.6 Insertion of suprapubic catheter

Key points

A suprapubic catheter is a tube that is inserted through the abdominal wall directly into the bladder. It is used as a method of temporary or long-term urinary diversion when catheterisation via the urethra is not possible or desired. It is used following urethral trauma, reconstructive procedures for epispadias or complex hypospadias, and in cases of posterior urethral valves. It is also used to carry out urodynamic studies in children.[1]

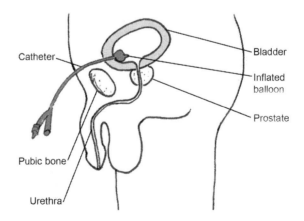

FIGURE 7.5 Insertion of suprapubic catheter.

Procedural considerations
- Usually general anaesthesia with local anaesthesia.
- Single dose of intravenous aminoglycoside antibiotic given at anaesthetic induction.[1]
- Length of stay depends on underlying diagnosis.
- Suprapubic catheter insertion requires a full bladder.
- Ultrasound is often used to aid insertion.
- Preassembled kits are usually used – these use the Seldinger technique or use a trocar, with the catheter placed either simultaneously with the trocar or through it.
- Local anaesthetic is infiltrated into the skin and fascial layers, 1–2 fingerbreadths above the pubic symphysis. Insertion technique depends on the kit used.

Postoperative considerations
- Mild transient haematuria is normal after suprapubic catheter insertion.
- If suprapubic catheterisation is required long term, the catheter must be changed every 3 to 4 months (depending on catheter type).

Additional considerations
- If a suprapubic catheter is inserted to divert urine following urethral or penile surgery then placement should be included in the consent for the main operation.
- Alternatives
  - Urethral catheterisation – this is usually used if possible. It carries risk of urethral injury, urethral stricture, urethritis or meatitis and urinary tract infection.[2]
  - Permanent urinary diversion.

CONSENT FORM
Name of procedure: Suprapubic catheter insertion
Benefits:
> Drainage of urine from bladder
> (The intended benefit is dependent on the indication for the suprapubic catheter.)

Risks:
> Overall minor complication rate of 5%[1]
> **General:**
> > Pain
> > Wound infection
> **Specific:**
> > Haematuria
> > Urinary tract infection: 7%[3]
> > Peritoneal irritation from urine leakage
> > Catheter dislodgement from bladder
> > Bladder stone formation (in the long term)
> > Bowel perforation
> > Bladder injury

Procedure involves: General and local anaesthesia

Key publications

O'Kelly TJ, Mathew A, Ross S, *et al*. Optimum method for urinary drainage in major abdominal surgery: a prospective randomized trial of suprapubic versus urethral catheterization. *Br J Surg*. 1995; **82**(10): 1367–8.[3]
- Prospective randomised trial.
- 57 adult patients undergoing abdominal surgery.
- 28 received a suprapubic and 29 a urethral catheter.
- Urinary sepsis occurred in three patients in each group.
- Urethral catheters caused pain in significantly more patients (urethral: 13, suprapubic: 2).

References
1 Wagner AA, Godley ML, Duffy PG, *et al*. A novel, inexpensive, double lumen suprapubic catheter for urodynamics. *J Urol*. 2004; **171**(3): 1277–9.
2 Rink RC, Cain MP. Urinary diversion. In: Belman AB, King LR, Kramer SA. *Clinical Pediatric Urology*. 4th ed. London: Taylor & Francis; 2002. pp. 491–528.
3 O'Kelly TJ, Mathew A, Ross S, *et al*. Optimum method for urinary drainage in major abdominal surgery: a prospective randomized trial of suprapubic versus urethral catheterization. *Br J Surg*. 1995; **82**(10): 1367–8.

7.7 Operative management of ingrowing toenails
Key points

Ingrowing toenails are common (approximately 10 000 cases/year in the UK[1]). They occur when the lateral margins of the nail penetrate the dermis due to improper fitting of the nail plate in the nail groove. This results in pain, inflammation and often infection and overgrowth of granulation tissue. The big toe is usually affected. The condition is observed in people of all ages but is most common in the second decade of life. Causes are thought to include wearing tight fitting shoes, hyperhidrosis, cutting nails too short or not cutting them straight.

Procedural considerations
- Day-case procedure.
- General/regional anaesthesia (digital nerve block).
- Tourniquet.

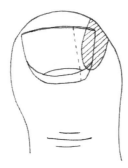

FIGURE 7.6 Operative management of ingrowing toenails.

- Wedge resection: incision made at base of nail fold. The nail is then cut longitudinally and the offending portion avulsed. The germinal matrix in this area is then eradicated either by surgical or chemical matrixectomy using phenol or NaOH.
- Zadek's procedure: two oblique incisions are made on the medial and lateral aspects of the toe over the matrical area. The entire nail matrix is removed.

Postoperative considerations
- Jelonet™ gauze and compression bandage.
- Keep the site dry.
- Keep foot elevated.
- No mobilisation for one day then limit weight bearing until healing has taken place.
- Topical antibiotics do not reduce the rate of postoperative infection or recurrence.[2,3]

Additional considerations
- Although not a complication, when performing a matrixectomy it is important to inform patients/parents that the nail will be permanently narrowed (wedge) or removed (Zadek's).
- If phenol is used, wound healing and return to activity are slower and postoperative infection rates are higher.[1,2,3]
- Alternative treatments and outcomes:
  - Conservative – elevating the edge of nail from the soft tissue and placement of a small pledget of cotton under the nail edge. Recurrence rate 5%–21%.[2,4] This is dependent on careful case selection.
  - Simple avulsion of the toenail – nail regrows with recurrence rate >50%.[2]

CONSENT FORM

Name of procedure: Wedge excision of nail and matrixectomy OR Zadek's procedure (removal of entire nail and matrixectomy)

Benefits:
  Relief of symptoms
  Treatment of ingrowing toenail to prevent recurrence

Risks:
  General:
  Bleeding
  Pain
  Specific:
  Infection – soft tissue (5.2%[2]), osteomyelitis (0.8%[2])
  Recurrence rate:
    Surgical matrixectomy: 20%–41%[2,3]
    Chemical matrixectomy: 1%–14%[2,3]

Procedure involves: General/regional anaesthesia

Key publications

Rounding C, Bloomfield S. Surgical treatments for ingrowing toenails. Cochrane Database Syst Rev. 2003; 1: CD001541.[1]
- Systematic review – nine randomised controlled trials comparing surgical management of ingrowing toenails included.

- Use of phenol with nail avulsion is more effective than excisional surgical procedures at preventing symptomatic recurrence.
- When performing a total or partial nail avulsion, the use of phenol dramatically reduced the rate of symptomatic recurrence (OR 0.07) but significantly increased the rate of postoperative infection (OR 5.69).

Bos AM, van Tilburg MW, van Sorge AA, *et al*. Randomized clinical trial of surgical technique and local antibiotics for ingrowing toenail. *Br J Surg*. 2007; **94**(3): 292–6.[3]
- Randomised controlled trial.
- 123 patients with ingrowing toenails, 117 in follow up. All had partial nail avulsion.
- Patients randomised to have excision of the matrix or application of phenol with or without local application antibiotics afterwards.
- Recurrence at 1 year was significantly less in phenol group (13.8%) than matrix excision group (40.7%).
- In terms of signs of infection, there was no significant difference between phenol and matrix excision.

References

1 Rounding C, Bloomfield S. Surgical treatments for ingrowing toenails. Cochrane Database Syst Rev. 2003; 1: CD001541.
2 Yang G, Yanchar NL, Lo AY, *et al*. Treatment of ingrown toenails in the pediatric population. *J Pediatr Surg*. 2008; **43**(5): 931–5
3 Bos AM, van Tilburg MW, van Sorge AA, *et al*. Randomized clinical trial of surgical technique and local antibiotics for ingrowing toenail. *Br J Surg*. 2007; **94**(3): 292–6.
4 Lazar L, Erez I, Katz S. A conservative treatment for ingrown toenails in children. *Pediatr Surg Int*. 1999; **15**(2): 121–2.

Plastic surgery

8.1 Excision of malignant skin lesion

Key points

The commonest malignant skin lesions are basal cell carcinomas (BCC), squamous cell carcinomas (SCC) and malignant melanomas (MM). Less common lesions include Merkel cell tumours, adnexal tumours and sarcomas.

Procedural considerations

* Local/regional/general anaesthesia – depends on size, location, age and co-morbidities.
* The extent of the lesion is marked with a skin marker under good lighting. An additional 'margin' of clinically normal skin is marked around this to allow for subclinical extension. The margin taken depends on the suspected diagnosis (specific guidelines are available).
* The marked lesion is generally extended in to an ellipse and placed within relaxed skin tension lines (if possible) to facilitate skin closure and allow for a less visible scar.
* Careful consideration must be given to the direction of excision of any possible malignant lesion as they may require a further and wider excision.

Postoperative considerations

* The majority of patients have small skin lesions and the procedure is undertaken as a day case. Inpatient stay may be required if the lesion is large and requires extensive excision and/or any reconstructive procedures, if there are any immediate postoperative complications (e.g. bleeding), or due to patient co-morbidities/social circumstances.
* An outpatient appointment is booked within a few weeks to discuss histology results and any further management.

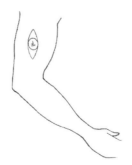

FIGURE 8.1 Excision of malignant skin lesion.

Additional considerations

Alternative treatments:

- No treatment: malignant lesions by nature will progress, invade surrounding structures and metastasise. The option of no treatment should be advised only if the patient is frail and has co-morbidities that make treatment modalities unsafe.
- BCC/SCC: surgical excision (including Mohs' micrographic surgery) is a highly effective treatment for BCC and SCC. Less aggressive surgical techniques (curettage and cautery, cryosurgery, carbon dioxide laser) and non-surgical techniques (topical immunotherapy, photodynamic therapy for BCC) are recommended only for low-risk disease and provided a confident clinical diagnosis has been made.[1,3] Radiotherapy is effective for primary and recurrent BCC, as adjuvant therapy, and for those unable to tolerate surgery.[1] There are no prospective randomised studies comparing different types of treatment for SCC.[3]
- MM: surgical excision is the definitive treatment for the primary lesion. The role of adjuvant therapy is yet to be established. Current studies do not suggest any survival benefit with adjuvant chemo or radiotherapy.[5]

CONSENT FORM

Name of procedure: Excision of suspected malignant lesion

Benefits:

Diagnosis and cure

If cure is not possible, excision may be undertaken for symptom control

Risks:

General:

Infection

Bleeding/haematoma

Adverse scarring (including hypertrophic/keloid scarring)

Specific:

Incomplete excision:

Basal cell carcinoma: 4.7%–7%[1]

Squamous cell carcinoma:

Lesions <2 cm: 5% with 4 mm margin[4]

(Lesions >2 cm/poorly differentiated/high risk sites require margins of 6 mm or more to obtain similar clearance rates)[4]

Malignant melanoma: these are excised with narrow (2 mm) margins initially as all histologically confirmed malignant melanomas require a wide local excision.

Recurrence: this depends on many factors including the location, size, histological type, thickness of the lesion, excision margins, perineural invasion (SCC) and ulceration (MM).

Basal cell carcinoma: <2%[2] at 5 years

Squamous cell carcinoma

Lesions <2 cm – local recurrence 7.4%[3]

Lesions >2 cm – local recurrence 15.2%[3]

Lesions >4 mm in thickness, or invading into subcutaneous tissue, or with perineural invasion, or if poorly differentiated, have a higher rate of recurrence[3]

Malignant melanoma[5]

Lesions <1 mm thick without ulceration: 5 year disease free survival >90%

Lesions <1 mm with ulceration, 1.01–2 mm (+/– ulceration), 2.01–4 mm without ulceration: 15–35% risk of recurrence (greatest risk at 2–4 yrs)

Lesions 2.01–4 mm with ulceration, >4 mm (+/– ulceration: 40–70% risk of recurrence (greatest risk at 2–4 yrs)

Further surgery: Wide local excision, lymph node surgery

Key publications

Telfer NR, Colver GB, Morton CA. Guidelines for the management of basal cell carcinoma. *Br J Dermatol*. 2008; **159**: 35–48.[1]

- These guidelines provide an overview of epidemiology, diagnosis, investigations and the evidence base for treatment options. Many treatment modalities available but very few randomised controlled trials comparing the different options.
- Surgical excision highly effective.
- Small (<2 cm) and well defined: 95% peripheral clearance with 4–5 mm margin.
- Large and morphoeic: >95% peripheral clearance with 13–15 mm margin.

Motley RJ, Preston PW, Lawrence CM. Multiprofessional guidelines for the management of the patient with primary cutaneous squamous cell carcinoma. *BJD*. 2009. (Update of the original guideline which appeared in *BJD*. 2002; **146**(1): 18–25.)[3]

- SCCs of the lip or ear, arising in non-sun exposed areas, more than 2 cm in diameter, more than 4 mm in depth, moderately or poorly differentiated, and in immunosuppressed patients, are considered high risk.
- Surgical excision is the general treatment of choice.

Marsden JR, Newton-Bishop JA, Burrows L, Cook M, Corrie PG, Cox NH, Gore ME, Lorigan P, MacKie R, Nathan P, Peach H, Powell B, Walker C. Revised UK guidelines for the management of cutaneous melanoma 2010. *British Journal of Dermatology*. DOI: 10.1111/j.1365-2133.2010.09883.x[5]

- Surgical excision margins should be 1 cm for MMs <1 mm, 1–2 cm for MMs 1.01–2 mm, 2-3 cm for MMs 2.1 mm and 3cm for MMs >4mm.
- Follow up: if the MM is <1 mm, with no ulceration and mitoses the patient should be seen 2 to 4 years in the first 12 months, then discharged. The rest should be followed up 3-monthly for 3 years and then 6-monthly to 5 years or annually to 10 years depending on the stage of melanoma.

References

1 Telfer NR, Colver GB, Morton CA. Guidelines for the management of basal cell carcinoma. *Br J Dermatol*. 2008; **159**: 35–48.
2 Griffiths RW, Suvarna SK, Stone J. Do basal cell carcinomas recur after complete conventional surgical excision? *Br J Plast Surg*. 2005; **58**: 795–805.
3 Motley RJ, Preston PW, Lawrence CM. Multiprofessional guidelines for the management of the patient with primary cutaneous squamous cell carcinoma 2009. *Update of the original guideline which appeared in BJD, Vol. 146, No. 1, January 2002 (p18-25)*.
4 Brodland DG, Zitelli JA. Surgical margins for excision of primary cutaneous squamous cell carcinoma. *J Am Acad Dermatol*. 1992; **27**. 241–8.

5 Marsden JR, Newton-Bishop JA, Burrows L, Cook M, Corrie PG, Cox NH, Gore ME, Lorigan P, MacKie R, Nathan P, Peach H, Powell B, Walker C. Revised UK guidelines for the management of cutaneous melanoma 2010. *British Journal of Dermatology.* DOI: 10.1111/j.1365-2133.2010.09883.x

8.2 Excision of sebaceous cyst
Key points
An epidermoid cyst (also known as an epidermal inclusion cyst or sebaceous cyst) is a common benign skin tumour, commonly found on the face, back, and chest. These cysts can arise due to blockage of pilosebaceous follicles or implantation/trapping of epidermal cells into the dermis along embryological fusion planes or due to trauma.[1] There is normally a channel through which the cyst communicates with the surface (punctum). Cysts are removed if they are symptomatic (discomfort, inflammation, infection, rupture and discharge) or for cosmetic reasons.

Procedural considerations
- Local anaesthesia.
- Skin crease excision with ellipse of skin including the punctum. Excision is made easier by grasping the skin with forceps whilst the cyst is dissected free from surrounding tissues. It is important to remove the entire epithelial lining to prevent recurrence.
- Specimen must always be sent for histology as it may masquerade as other lesions for example leiomyosarcoma or sebaceous carcinoma.

Postoperative considerations
- Light dressing.

Additional considerations
Alternative treatments:
- No treatment
  - Epidermoid cysts are normally slow growing and asymptomatic. Most cysts do not require any treatment.
- Medical treatment
  - Intralesional injection of triamcinolone may help decrease inflammation. Antibiotics and incision and drainage are required if the cyst is infected. Once the infection has resolved further surgery is performed to remove the entire cyst.
- Surgical treatment – three techniques exist
  - The traditional wide elliptical excision (described above) is the gold standard and most commonly performed.

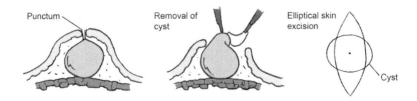

FIGURE 8.2 Excision of sebaceous cyst.

- Minimal excision and punch biopsy excision are alternative techniques that involve either a 3 mm incision or dermal punch, through which the cyst contents and wall are removed via kneading or lateral pressure. The wound may be closed with sutures or left open to heal.
- Advantages reported include minimal bleeding, faster healing and less scarring. In a series of 302 patients undergoing minimal excision surgery the recurrence rate was reported as 0.66% over an 18-month follow-up period.[2] Another retrospective review of 646 patients who underwent punch excision over a 9-year period revealed a recurrence rate of <10%.[3]
- There are no randomised controlled studies to compare the outcomes of the three techniques. A trial is on the way for comparison of excision vs. punch incision.[4]

Other treatments: carbon dioxide laser has been used to treat epidermoid cysts.[5]

CONSENT FORM
Name of procedure: Excision of sebaceous cyst
Benefits:
Cure and relief of symptoms
Improved cosmesis
Risks:
General:
Infection – no published figures available
Bleeding
Adverse scarring (including hypertrophic/keloid scars)
Specific:
Recurrence – low if cyst fully excised
Further surgery – for recurrence or if histology proves alternative pathology
Procedure involves: Local/general anaesthesia (if large)

Key publications

Lee HE, Yang CH, Chen CH, *et al.* Comparison of the surgical outcomes of punch incision and elliptical excision in treating epidermal inclusion cysts: a prospective, randomized study. *Dermatol Surg.* 2006; **32**(4): 520–56.[6]

- 60 patients with non-infected cysts were randomised to have either punch incision or elliptical incision by a single dermatologist.
- Mean wound lengths were 0.73 cm and 2.34 cm respectively.
- Mean operative time was significantly shorter in the punch group (12.7 minutes) compared with the surgical group (21.6 minutes) (p<0.001).
- No significant difference in the recurrence rate (1/31 in the punch biopsy group, 0/29 in the wide excision group).
- Removal of cysts larger than 2 cm took longer with the punch biopsy technique.
- The main shortcomings include small study group and short follow-up period. No larger studies are currently available.

References.

1 Mathes SJ, and Hentz VR, editors. *Plastic Surgery, Vol. 5.* 2nd ed. Philadelphia, PA: Saunders, 2006; p. 255.
2 Klin B, Ashkenazi H. Sebaceous cyst excision with minimal surgery. *Am Fam Physician.* 1990; **41**(6): 1746–8.

3 Mehrabi D, Leonhardt JM, Brodell RT. Removal of keratinous and pilar cysts with the punch incision technique: analysis of surgical outcomes. *Dermatol Surg.* 2002; **28**: 673–7.

4 Comparison of excision versus punch incision in the treatment of epidermal cysts. http://clinicaltrials.gov/ct2/show/NCT00165958?term=Epidermoid+cyst&rank=1 (accessed 13 June 2010).

5 Reynolds N, Kenealy J. Use of a carbon dioxide laser in the treatment of multiple epidermoid cysts. *Br J Plast Surg.* 2002; **55**(3): 260.

6 Lee HE, Yang CH, Chen CH, *et al.* Comparison of the surgical outcomes of punch incision and elliptical excision in treating epidermal inclusion cysts: a prospective, randomized study. *Dermatol Surg.* 2006; **32**(4): 520–5.

8.3 Skin grafting
Key points
A skin graft is a piece of skin that is moved from one body part to another without its blood supply. It is indicated for defects that cannot be closed primarily. The graft may include all layers of epidermis and dermis (full-thickness skin graft, FTSG) or epidermis and only part of the dermis (split skin graft, SSG). The thicker the dermal component, the more characteristics of normal skin are maintained following grafting. A skin graft is reliant on establishing a new blood supply at the recipient site and thus requires a vascularised bed.

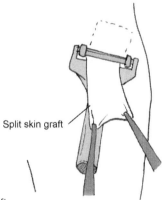

Split skin graft

FIGURE 8.3A Split skin graft.

Procedural considerations
- Local/regional/general anaesthesia – depends on size.
- SSG: a powered dermatome or skin graft knife can be used for harvest. Although it can be harvested from anywhere, common donor sites include the lateral or medial thigh, scalp and back. The donor site heals by epithelialisation – the scar is the size of the graft taken. The graft is often meshed (allowing expansion) and secured to the recipient site with tissue glue, staples or sutures.
- FTSG: common sites include pre- or postauricular skin, supraclavicular skin, antecubital fossa, medial arm and groin. The donor site is closed directly. The graft is secured with sutures with or without a tie-over dressing.

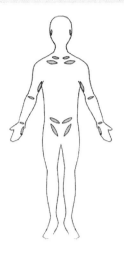

FIGURE 8.3B Full-thickness skin graft donor sites.

- In the past any excess grafts have been saved for delayed grafting. Since September 2006, the UK Human Tissue Act dictates that storing any tissue part for transplantation is not permitted without a licence. However, skin may be stored for up to 48 hours without the need for a licence.[1]

Postoperative considerations
- Bulky dressings may be used. The graft must be protected from any shearing forces. A splint may be applied to immobilise any joints that contribute towards movement of the graft.
- A graft check is often performed between 3 and 14 days. Donor-site dressings are kept on for up to 2 weeks for SSGs.

Additional considerations
Alternative treatments:
- Healing by secondary intention
  - If the defect is small, it may be allowed to heal by secondary intention. If the patient is unfit for or does not want surgery, larger defects may also be allowed to heal by this method. Patients should be advised regarding the long healing time, need for repeated dressing changes, and possibility of infection.
- Local flaps
  - Flaps are normally performed if the defect does not have a vascularised bed. However, in certain locations flaps may be preferred instead of skin grafts as they can offer better cosmesis, e.g. on the face, but they carry risks of failure, bulk and pincushioning. Caution must be observed before using a local flap for reconstruction of a defect following excision of a possibly malignant lesion, as further surgical options may be compromised.
- Skin substitutes
  - Cultured epithelial autografts (CEA): cultured epithelial cells require a biopsy from the patient followed by growth of the cells in culture. They take a few weeks to form confluent sheets and they are fragile and sensitive to infection. CEA may have an important role in the treatment of major burns but further research is required.[2]

- Allografts and xenografts
  - Temporary skin substitutes that act as biologic dressings only. They are eventually rejected by the patient's immune system, and need to be replaced with definitive skin coverage. In addition, cost and the possibility of disease transmission are factors to consider with such substitutes.
- Biosynthetic materials
  - There are many commercially available biosynthetic materials that can act as temporary epidermal and/or dermal substitutes. They do not require a donor site, and so decrease metabolic demands on the patient.[3] Dermal analogues may improve the appearance of skin grafts, thus avoiding the need for a skin flap in an area of aesthetic concern.

CONSENT FORM

Name of procedure: Reconstruction of skin defect with split/full-thickness skin graft

Benefits:

Improve healing

Risks:

General:

Infection

Bleeding/haematoma

Specific:

Graft failure (partial or complete)

May be related to haematoma/seroma under graft,[4] infection (up to 23.5%),[8] poor vascular bed, shearing forces, technical problems.

Group A beta-haemolytic *Streptococcus* and *Pseudomonas aeruginosa* are associated with graft failure.

Seroma

Adverse scarring including scar at donor site

Scar contracture[5]

Hypo/hyperpigmentation

SSGs are darker than FTSGs from the same donor site[5]

Grafts taken from brunettes darken, while those from blondes lighten[5]

Immediately after harvesting, a skin graft blanches from circulatory interruption. The subsequent loss of melanoblast content causes profound alteration in the ratio of pigment-producing to non-pigment-producing cells in the graft.[7]

Poor sensitivity of graft[6]

Procedure involves: Local/regional/general anaesthesia

Key publications

Unal S, Ersoz G, Demirkan F, Arslan E, Tütüncü N, Sari A. Analysis of skin-graft loss due to infection: infection-related graft loss. *Ann Plast Surg.* 2005 Jul; **55**(1): 102–6.[8]

- Prospective study examining the rate of skin graft loss due to infection.
- 132 patients with soft tossue defects due to trauma, vascular ulcers, burns, flap donor sites were reconstructed with full or split-thickness skin grafts in adequately prepared wound-beds.
- Graft loss due to infection: 31 patients (23.5%).

- *Pseudomonas aeruginosa* was the main causative organism (58.1% of failed grafts).
- The majority of failed grafts were in patients with vascular ulcers and burns.
- The authors also found that full-thickness grafts were more resistant to infection than split-thickness grafts.

References

1 Patel AJK. Implications of the Human Tissue Act (2004) on tissue storage for UK plastic surgeons. *J Plast Reconstr Aesthet Surg.* 2009; **62**(8): 983–5.
2 Wood FM, Kolybaba ML, Allen P. The use of cultured epithelial autograft in the treatment of major burn injuries: a critical review of the literature. *Burns.* 2006; **32**(4): 395–401.
3 Mathes SJ. *Plastic Surgery.* 2nd ed. Philadelphia, PA: Saunders; 2006.
4 Flowers RS. Unexpected postoperative problems in skin grafting. *Surg Clin North Am.* 1970; **50**: 439–56.
5 Kelton PL. Skin grafts and skin substitutes. *Select Read Plast Surg.* 1999; **9**(1): 1–24.
6 Stella M, Calcagni M, Teich-Alasia S, *et al.* Sensory endings in skin grafts and scars after extensive burns. *Burns.* 1994; **20**(6): 491–5.
7 Conway H, Sedar J. Report of the loss of pigment in full thickness autoplastic skin grafts in the mouse. *Plast Reconstr Surg.* 1956; **18**: 30.
8 Unal S, Ersoz G, Demirkan F, Arslan E, Tütüncü N, Sari A. Analysis of skin-graft loss due to infection: infection-related graft loss. *Ann Plast Surg.* 2005 Jul; **55**(1): 102–6.

8.4 Ganglion excision

Key points

A ganglion is a cyst filled with clear viscous jelly-like mucinous material made up of glucosamine, albumin, globulin, and a high concentration of hyaluronic acid.[1] Commonly found on the dorsal (60%–70%) or volar (18%–20%) aspect of the wrist,[2] it is attached to the joint capsule, tendon or tendon sheath. Other locations include the flexor tendon sheath, distal interphalangeal joint (DIPJ) (also known as a mucous cyst), and proximal interphalangeal joint (PIPJ).

Procedural considerations

- Method may vary according to location of ganglion.
- Day-case procedure.
- General/regional anaesthesia.
- Arm tourniquet.
- A transverse incision is made over the ganglion, followed by dissection to expose the ganglion. Branches of dorsal radial and ulnar sensory nerves, and radial artery are

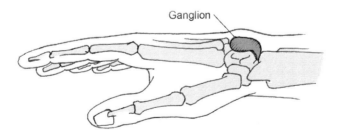

FIGURE 8.4 Ganglion cyst.

identified and protected. The ganglion is excised with its capsular attachments and the wound is then closed.

Postoperative considerations
- Small dressing.
- Elevation.
- Mobilise as comfort allows.

Additional considerations
Alternative treatments and outcomes:
- No treatment
  - Spontaneous resolution if untreated – volar 53%[3], dorsal 42%.[4]
- Aspiration +/– steroid injection
  - Recurrence rate – volar 47%[3], dorsal 58%.[4]
  - A prospective randomised study showed no benefit of steroid infiltration over simple aspiration.[5]
- Aspiration and hyaluronidase acid injection
  - Recurrence rate – 77%.[6]
- Arthroscopic resection: complication and recurrence rates similar to open resection.[7,8]

Ganglions in children have a particularly high spontaneous resolution rate.[9]

Scapho-lunate instability following excision of dorsal wrist ganglion: although isolated reports suggest this can be a complication, a review of 91 patients post ganglionectomy suggests this is not the case.[10]

CONSENT FORM

Name of procedure: Excision of ganglion cyst from (left/right) anatomical location

Benefits:
 Relief of symptoms (pain, stiffness, cosmesis)

Risks:
 Overall: 8%[2]
 General:
  Infection
  Bleeding/haematoma
  Wound dehiscence
  Adverse scarring – including hypertrophic/keloid scar: 1%[2]
  Scar tenderness: 4%[2]
  Numbness: 3%[2]
 Specific:
  Neurovascular injury
   Radial artery injury in volar wrist ganglion excision
   Injury to palmar cutaneous nerve of median nerve in volar wrist ganglion: 20%[11]
  Recurrence
   Rate – volar wrist 42%[1], dorsal wrist 39%[2]
  Wrist stiffness (dorsal wrist ganglion) – may worsen postop[2]

> For mucous cyst
> Extensor lag
> Joint stiffness
> Nail plate deformity
> Deviation of distal interphalangeal joint
> **Procedure involves:** General and/or regional anaesthesia

Key publications

Dias J, Buch K. Palmar wrist ganglion: does intervention improve outcome? A prospective study of the natural history and patient-reported treatment outcomes. *J Hand Surg Br.* 2003; **28**(2): 172–6.[3]
- Prospective cohort study of 155 patients.
- 2- and 5-year follow-up.
- No significant difference in recurrence rate between aspiration and excision.
- No difference in symptoms was found, whether the palmar wrist ganglion was excised, aspirated or left alone.
- 20% complication rate with surgery.

Dias JJ, Dhukaram V, Kumar P. The natural history of untreated dorsal wrist ganglia and patient reported outcome 6 years after intervention. *J Hand Surg Eur.* 2007; **32**(5): 502–8.[4]
- Prospective cohort study of 236 patients.
- Postal questionnaire at a mean of 70 months.
- Neither excision nor aspiration provided significant long-term benefit over no treatment.
- 8% complication rate with surgery.

References

1 Soren A. Pathogenesis and treatment of ganglion. *Clin Orthop.* 1966; **48**: 173–9.
2 Angelides AC. Ganglions of the hand and wrist. In: Green DP, Hotchkiss RN, Pederson WC, editors. *Operative Hand Surgery, Vol 2.* 4th ed. New York: Churchill Livingstone; 1999. pp. 2171–83.
3 Dias J, Buch K. Palmar wrist ganglion: does intervention improve outcome? – a prospective study of the natural history and patient-reported treatment outcomes. *J Hand Surg Br.* 2003; **28**(2): 172–6.
4 Dias JJ, Dhukaram V, Kumar P. The natural history of untreated dorsal wrist ganglia and patient reported outcome 6 years after intervention. *J Hand Surg Eur.* 2007; **32**(5): 502–8.
5 Varley GW, Needoff M, Davis TR, *et al.* Conservative management of wrist ganglia: aspiration versus steroid infiltration. *J Hand Surg.* 1997; **22**(5): 636–7.
6 Jagers Op Akkerhuis M, Van Der Heijden M, Brink PR. Hyaluronidase versus surgical excision of ganglia: a prospective, randomized clinical trial. *J Hand Surg Br.* 2002; **27**(3): 256–8.
7 Dumontier C, Chaumeil G, Chassat R, *et al.* Arthroscopic treatment of dorsal wrist ganglia. *Chir Main.* 2006; **25**(Suppl. 1): S214–20.
8 Edwards SG, Johansen JA. Prospective outcomes and associations of wrist ganglion cysts resected arthroscopically. *J Hand Surg Am.* 2009; **34**(3): 395–400.
9 Rosson JW, Walker G. The natural history of ganglia in children. *J Bone Joint Surg Br.* 1989; **71**: 707–8.
10 Kivett WF, Wood FM, Rauscher GE, *et al.* Does ganglionectomy destabilize the wrist over the long-term? *Ann Plast Surg.* 1996; **36**(5): 466–8.

11 Jacobs LG, Govaers KJ. The volar wrist ganglion: just a simple cyst? *J Hand Surgery Br.* 1990; **15**: 342–6.

8.5 Carpal tunnel decompression

Key points

Carpal tunnel syndrome is the most common upper limb compression neuropathy. It is considered to be a compressive neuropathy of the median nerve as it courses through the carpal tunnel. Non-surgical treatment is reserved for mild to moderate disease.[1] Decompression of the median nerve is considered the standard surgical treatment for carpal tunnel syndrome (CTS). Surgery involves release of the transverse carpal ligament to increase the canal volume and reduce pressure on the nerve.

Procedural considerations

- Median nerve block at wrist/brachial block/general anaesthesia.
- An arm tourniquet may be used. Alternatively, using adrenaline with the local anaesthetic permits surgery without the use of a tourniquet.
- A 2–3 cm longitudinal incision in line with radial border of fourth ray is made over the carpal tunnel. Sharp dissection is undertaken through skin, subcutaneous fat and palmar aponeurosis. The transverse carpal tunnel ligament is identified and incised longitudinally under direct vision. Care must be taken to avoid injury to the recurrent branch of the median nerve (variable anatomy). The skin is closed with non-absorbable sutures.

Postoperative considerations

- Elevate in high arm sling.
- Day-case procedure.
- Mobilise as soon as possible, hand therapy.
- Removal of sutures in 10–14 days.

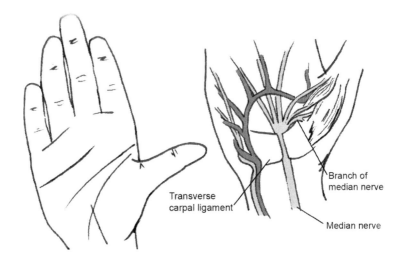

FIGURE 8.5 Open carpal tunnel release (OCTR).

Additional considerations

Alternative treatments:

- Non-surgical treatment
  - A recent Cochrane review[2] found some evidence of short-term benefit from oral steroids, splinting/hand braces, ultrasound and carpal bone mobilisation (movement of the bones and tissues in the wrist). Evidence for ergonomic keyboards and vitamin B6 is unclear. Studies have not shown benefit from diuretics, non-steroidal anti-inflammatory drugs, magnets, laser acupuncture, exercise or chiropractic.
  - Steroid injection: local steroid injection into the carpal tunnel can provide better symptom relief than placebo, at 1 month. No symptomatic relief beyond 1 month has been demonstrated. Two injections do not provide any benefit over one.[4]
  - A further Cochrane review assessing surgical vs. non-surgical treatment (splinting, steroid injections) favoured surgical treatment. The review found that a significant proportion of people treated medically will require surgery while the risk of reoperation in surgically treated people is low.[3]
- Endoscopic carpal tunnel release (ECTR)
  - The advantages of this procedure lie in the transverse carpal ligament being released from inside, thus leaving intact all the structures superficial to the tunnel. This decreases postoperative morbidity and allows quicker return to work. Symptomatic relief and functional scores post are similar to open relief[5] with few complications (0.19% major complication rate[6]).

CONSENT FORM

Name of procedure: Carpal tunnel decompression
Benefits:
      Improve symptoms
      Prevent worsening of symptoms
      Improve hand function
Risks:
      Overall complication rate: 12%[10]
General:
      Infection: 2.5%[5]
      Bleeding
Specific:
Major: structural damage to nerve, artery or tendon: 0.49%[6]
      Nerve injury
            Median nerve[9]
            Recurrent branch of median nerve
            Palmar cutaneous branch of median nerve (12.5% cross carpal tunnel[11])
            Ulnar nerve – deep motor branch: 1.5%[7,12]
            Digital nerve
      Vascular – superficial palmar arch
      Tendon – bowstringing of digital flexor tendon: 1.5%[7]
Minor:
      Pillar pain: pain in the thenar or hypothenar areas may be due to a variety of factors – scar sensitivity, neuromas of cutaneous nerve endings, changes

in carpal arch dynamics or thenar and hypothenar muscle origins, and/
or decreased median nerve gliding.
Chronic regional pain syndrome: 5.7[5]
Adverse scarring/scar sensitivity: 8%[5]
Wound dehiscence: 3%[7]
Persistence of symptoms/incomplete release: 2.6%[5]
    (Persistent symptoms may be because of untreated space-occupying
        lesions in the carpal tunnel, such as a ganglion, other tumour, dis-
        placed lunate, inflamed flexor tenosynovium, or a gouty tophus.)
Repeat surgery: 1.4%[5]
Recurrence: 7%[8]
Procedure involves: Local/regional/general anaesthesia

Key publications

Scholten RJPM, Mink van der Molen A, Uitdehaag BMJ, *et al*. Surgical treatment options for carpal tunnel syndrome. Cochrane Database Syst Rev. 2007; 4: CD003905.[5]
- Systematic review of randomised controlled trials which compared the short-term and long-term efficacies of the various surgical treatments.
- 41 studies included 16 studies comparing OCTR vs. ECTR.
- No significant difference in overall improvement, symptom severity or functional status in the short- or long-term between the two. One study found a significant decrease in pain scores at 12 months with ECTR.
- Three studies found that the time to return to work was significantly less (average 6 days) with ECTR.
- No major complications leading to permanent injury in either group.
- ECTR gives more transient nerve problems (e.g. neurapraxia, numbness, paraesthesiae).
- OCTR more wound problems (e.g. infection, hypertrophic scarring, scar tenderness).
- Repeated surgery was needed in 12 out of 513 ECTR procedures vs. 5 out of 370 OCTR procedures – relative risk of 1.2 in favour of OCTR.
- None of the existing alternatives to standard open carpal tunnel release offered significantly better relief from symptoms in the short- or long-term.

Braun RM, Rechnic M, Fowler E. Complications related to carpal tunnel release. *Hand Clin*. 2002; **18**: 347–57.[13]
- Review article looking at complications of carpal tunnel surgery.
- The article discusses nerve injury including palmar cutaneous nerve, the median motor branch, and the median nerve.
- The article describes recurrent scar formation as the most commonly encountered complication following carpal tunnel release. The authors also discuss general complications including complex regional pain syndrome.

References

1 Duncan KH, Lewis RC, Foreman KA, *et al*. Treatment of carpal tunnel syndrome by members of the American Society for Surgery of the Hand: results of a questionnaire. *J Hand Surg Am*. 1987; **12**(3): 384–91.
2 O'Connor D, Marshall SC, Massy-Westropp N. Non-surgical treatment (other than steroid injection) for carpal tunnel syndrome. Cochrane Database Syst Rev. 2003; 1: CD003219.

3 Verdugo RJ, Salinas RA, Castillo JL, *et al.* Surgical versus non-surgical treatment for carpal tunnel syndrome. Cochrane Database Syst Rev. 2008; 4: CD001552.
4 Marshall SC, Tardif G, Ashworth NL. Local corticosteroid injection for carpal tunnel syndrome. Cochrane Database Syst Rev. 2007; 2: CD001554.
5 Scholten RJPM, Mink van der Molen A, Uitdehaag BMJ, *et al.* Surgical treatment options for carpal tunnel syndrome. Cochrane Database Syst Rev. 2007; 4: CD003905.
6 Benson LS, Bare AA, Nagle DJ, *et al.* Complications of endoscopic and open carpal tunnel release. *Arthroscopy.* 2006; **22**(9): 919–24.
7 Agee JM, McCarroll HR Jr, Tortosa RD, *et al.* Endoscopic release of the carpal tunnel: a randomized prospective multicenter study. *J Hand Surg Am.* 1992; **17**(6): 987–95.
8 Eichhorn J, Dieterich K. Open versus endoscopic carpal tunnel release: results of a prospective study. *Chirurg Praxis.* 2003; **61**(2): 279–83.
9 Cartotto RC, McCabe S, Mackinnon SE. Two devastating complications of carpal tunnel surgery. *Ann Plast Surg.* 1992; **28**: 472.
10 MacDonald RI, Lichman DM, Hanlon JJ, *et al.* Complications of surgical release for carpal tunnel syndrome. *J Hand Surg Am.* 1978; **3**: 70–6.
11 Born T, Mahoney J. Cutaneous distribution of the ulnar nerve in the palm: does it cross the incision used in carpal tunnel release? *Ann Plast Surg.* 1995; **35**: 23–5.
12 Yoong P, Fattah A, Flemming AS. *Indian J Plast Surg.* 2008; **41**(1): 73–5.
13 Braun RM, Rechnic M, Fowler E. Complications related to carpal tunnel release. *Hand Clin.* 2002; **18**: 347–57.

8.6 Release of trigger finger
Key points
A mismatch between the size of the flexor tendon and pulley at the entrance to the tendon sheath restricts gliding of the tendon. Thus a triggering digit (often painful), or a digit locked in flexion ensues. Co-morbid conditions such as diabetes mellitus affect response to treatment.[1]

Surgical treatment involves release of the A1 pulley of the affected tendon sheath, thus allowing the tendon to glide smoothly. Surgery is indicated if conservative management and steroid injection has failed.

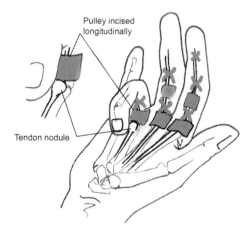

Pulley incised longitudinally

Tendon nodule

FIGURE 8.6 Release of trigger finger.

Procedural considerations
- Local/regional anaesthesia.
- A longitudinal, transverse or oblique incision is made over the A1 pulley at the base of the finger. The A1 pulley is identified and incised longitudinally. The finger is tested to make sure there is no restriction to movement. Neurovascular bundles on either side of the pulley must be protected (especially the radial digital nerve of the thumb and index finger).[1] Care must also be taken not to injure the A2 pulley.
- Surgical release is not recommended in patients with rheumatoid arthritis as this can make their ulnar drift worse. These patients benefit from tenosynovectomy.

Postoperative considerations
- Small dressing.
- Mobilise as comfort allows.
- Physiotherapy may be required for the elderly or those with longstanding triggering or fixed flexion contractures.

Additional considerations
Alternative treatments:
- Activity modification
  - Spontaneous resolution may occur with activity modification, if a specific triggering activity can be identified. Non-steroidal anti-inflammatory drugs can be used as an adjunct.[1]
- Splinting
  - Splinting (of the MCPJ at 10–15° flexion for 6 weeks) can be considered in patients with mild triggering who do not want steroid injection or surgery.[1] However, there are few studies that look at splinting in isolation. Splinting is often combined with steroid injection or surgery.
- Steroid injection
  - Long-acting steroid injection into the tendon sheath has been used with success rates of 60% to 92% with up to three injections in providing long-term relief of symptoms.[2] However, a recent prospective study found a 56% recurrence rate at 1 year after steroid injection.[3] Complications are rare (fat necrosis, skin depigmentation, tendon atrophy). Success rates are better if relatively recent onset of symptoms (<4 months), single digit involvement, and discrete palpable nodule.[2] Poorer outcome has been observed in patients with diabetes (50% success),[4] younger age,[3] involvement of multiple digits,[2,3] history of other tendinopathies,[3] diffuse disease(48% success)[2] and symptoms present for longer than 6 months.[2]
- Percutaneous trigger finger release
  - This is performed under local anaesthesia with a 18 gauge needle (or especially designed hook, blade or knife) to release the A1 pulley. Incomplete release and safety of the digital nerves are the main concerns with this procedure – 74%–100% success rates have been reported with minimal complications.[5,6,9] Scarring of the flexor tendon under the pulley has also been noted, leading to painful tenosynovitis. However, this is temporary with no long-term consequences.[1]
- Other techniques
  - More extensive procedures may be required in select cases,[1] e.g. ulnar superficialis slip resection, reduction flexor tenoplasty, A3 pulley release, tenosynovectomy.

CONSENT FORM

Name of procedure: Release of trigger finger

Benefits:

 Relief of symptoms

Risks:

 General:

  Infection

  Bleeding

  Scar tenderness – generally temporary

 Specific:

  Continued triggering/incomplete release: 3%[8]

  Recurrence: 1.8%[9]

  Stiffness

  Digital nerve injury (altered sensation) – infrequent – more likely in the thumb or index finger.[1]

  Bowstringing – if A2 pulley accidentally cut resulting in altered digital function and loss of full flexion/extension – rare.[7]

Procedure involves: General and/or regional anaesthesia

Key publications

Ryzewicz M, Wolf JM. Trigger digits: principles, management, and complications. *J Hand Surg Am.* 2006; **31**(1): 135–46.[1]

- This is a review article detailing the pathomechanics, risk factors, various treatments and evidence relating to treatment modalities.
- Appropriate treatment is based on understanding the location and nature of the mismatch.
- Activity modification, anti-inflammatory medication, splinting, corticosteroid injection, and open and percutaneous A1 pulley are all treatment options.
- Patients with co-morbid conditions may require different treatment options.

Gilberts EC, Beekman WH, Stevens HJ, *et al.* Prospective randomized trial of open versus percutaneous surgery for trigger digits. *J Hand Surg Am.* 2001; **26**(3): 497–500.[9]

- 100 trigger digits (96 patients) were randomised to either open (n=46) or percutaneous (n=54) surgical release.
- 98% success with open surgical technique, and 100% success with percutaneous technique.
- Mean operation time was significantly longer (11 vs. 7 minutes) using the open technique.
- Mean duration of postoperative pain (3.1 vs. 5.7 days), and time to recovery of motor function (7 vs. 18 days after the procedure) and time to return to work (3.9 vs. 7.5 days) were significantly shorter for patients treated with the percutaneous method.
- No serious complications were observed in either group.

References

1 Ryzewicz M, Wolf JM. Trigger digits: principles, management, and complications. *J Hand Surg Am.* 2006; **31**(1): 135–46.

2 Freiberg A, Mulholland RS, Levine R. Non-operative treatment of trigger fingers and thumbs. *J Hand Surg Am.* 1989; **14**(3): 553–8.

3 Rozental TD, Zurakowski D, Blazar PE. Trigger finger: prognostic indicators of recurrence following corticosteroid injection. *J Bone Joint Surg Am.* 2008; **90**(8): 1665–72.

4 Griggs SM, Weiss AP, Lane LB, *et al.* Treatment of trigger fingers in patients with diabetes mellitus. *J Hand Surg Am.* 1995; **20**(5): 787–9.

5 Eastwood DM, Gupta KJ, Johnson DP. Percutaneous release of the trigger finger: an office procedure. *J Hand Surg Am.* 1992; **17**(1): 114–7.

6 Pope DF, Wolfe SW. Safety and efficacy of percutaneous trigger finger release. *J Hand Surg Am.* 1995; **20**(2): 280–3.

7 Heithoff SJ, Millender LH, Helman J. Bowstringing as a complication of trigger finger release. *J Hand Surg Am.* 1988; **13**(4): 567–70.

8 Turowski GA, Zdankiewicz PD, Thomson JG. The results of surgical treatment of trigger finger. *J Hand Surg Am.* 1997; **22**(1):145–9.

9 Gilberts EC, Beekman WH, Stevens HJ, *et al.* Prospective randomized trial of open versus percutaneous surgery for trigger digits. *J Hand Surg Am.* 2001; **26**(3): 497–500.

8.7 Extensor tendon repair

Key points

Extensor tendon lacerations are common in patients who have sustained hand trauma. These patients require extensive rehabilitation and may need subsequent surgery.[1] Primary suture repair is recommended for acute injuries.[2]

There are many methods of primary tendon repair and postoperative rehabilitation. The methods chosen depend on the level and nature of injury, patient cooperation with treatment regime, surgeon's preference and skills, availability of hand therapists. The aim of repair is to provide adhesion free, smooth gliding of the tendon in its sheath, thus restoring function.

Procedural considerations

- General/regional/local anaesthesia – depends on location and other injuries.
- Under tourniquet control, the initial wound from trauma is explored and extended as required for appropriate exposure. Retrieval of the proximal tendon stump may require extension of the skin incision. Care must be taken to protect neurovascular, ligamentous and other musculotendinous structures.
- All other structures are assessed and repaired as necessary (e.g. fracture fixation and neurovascular repair).
- The distal and proximal ends of the tendon are identified. Once the proximal end has been retrieved and the two ends approximated, the repair is performed (core

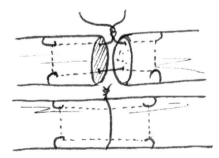

FIGURE 8.7 A method of tendon repair (modified Kessler).

and epitendinous where possible). The technique, type and number of sutures vary enormously. Multistrand repair is recommended.
- Once the wound is closed the digit or hand is immobilised in a splint.

Postoperative considerations
- Elevation.
- Postoperative rehabilitation contributes greatly towards long-term outcome. Early active motion is recommended in cooperative adult patients to minimise adhesion formation. The individual regimes vary.[2]
- Full use of the hand may not be possible for up to 12 weeks from repair– patients should be warned of this at the time of consent as it will affect work, sporting activities. Driving should be possible from 8 weeks.

Additional considerations
A detailed discussion should take place with the patient regarding tendon repair, postoperative hand therapy and variability of functional outcome.
Alternative treatments:
- Non-treatment
  - Non-treatment of a partial laceration (>60%) may lead to entrapment, triggering and rupture.
  - Non-treatment of a complete laceration will lead to permanent loss of function of that tendon, with resulting flexion or extension deformity of the finger. This may be appropriate in patients with pre-existing disease or co-morbidities where functional gain would be minimal.
  - Partial lacerations of <60% may not require repair and repair may lead to decreased tensile strength.[3]
  - A repair may be inappropriate for patients who are unwilling to cooperate with the postoperative rehabilitation regime or be immobilised in a splint.
- Other procedures – tendon grafts or staged reconstruction may be required for complicated injuries or late presentations.

CONSENT FORM
Name of procedure: Extensor tendon repair (state which finger)
Benefits:
   Improve function or restore function
Risks:
   General:
      Infection
      Bleeding
      Wound dehiscence
      Adverse scarring (inc. hypertrophic/keloid)
      Scar tenderness/numbness
      Anaesthetic complications
   Specific:
      Adhesions
      Rupture of repair
      Loss of flexion/extension[4]
      Joint contractures – DIPJ/PIPJ[5]

Stiffness
Neurovascular injury
Tendon graft
Further surgery (tenolysis, staged reconstruction)
Complex regional pain syndrome
Procedure involves: General and/or regional/local anaesthesia

Key publications
Newport ML, Blair WF, Steyers CM Jr. Long-term results of extensor tendon repair. *J Hand Surg Am.* 1990; **15**(6): 961–6.[4]
- Retrospective review of 62 patients with 101 extensor tendon injuries.
- 60% had associated other injuries (fractures, dislocations, joint capsule, flexor tendon).
- A static splinting regime post injury was used for the majority.
- 65% good/excellent results in patients without other injuries.
- 45% good/excellent in patients with other injuries.
- Outcome is worse in more distal extensor injuries.
- Loss of flexion is a greater than loss of extension in extensor tendon injuries.

References
1 Mathes SJ. *Plastic Surgery.* 2nd ed. Philadelphia, PA: Saunders; 2006.
2 *Selected Readings in Plastic Surgery.* Hand IV: Extensor tendons, Dupuytren's disease and rheumatoid arthritis. **9**(35).
3 *Selected Readings in Plastic Surgery.* Hand III: Flexor tendons. **9**(34).
4 Newport ML, Blair WF, Steyers CM Jr. Long-term results of extensor tendon repair. *J Hand Surg Am.* 1990; **15**(6): 961–6.
5 Su BW. Device for zone-II flexor tendon repair: a multicenter, randomized, blinded, clinical trial. *J Bone Joint Surg Am.* 2005; **87**: 923–35.

8.8 Peripheral nerve repair
Key points
Peripheral nerves can be injured, resulting in loss of motor or sensory function, or both. After a latent period, regeneration starts and the proximal end forms a growth cone. Under guidance of growth factors, branches from this enter the Schwann cell scar and find endoneurial tubes to continue down towards the target end organ. This process is facilitated by approximation of the proximal and distal ends by performing an end-to-end primary repair. Microsuture repair is the gold standard.

Procedural considerations
- Local/regional/general anaesthesia – depends on site and other associated injuries requiring surgery.
- Debate continues regarding the optimal technique of microsurgical neural repair. Epineural repair is generally recommended. However, in a prospective clinical study, no significant differences were observed between fascicular repair and epineural repair.[1]
- It should be a tension-free repair with minimal gapping. A nerve graft maybe

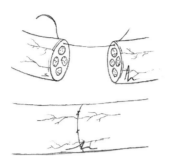

FIGURE 8.8 Epineurial repair of peripheral nerve.

required if there is segmental loss. Alternatively, a nerve conduit may be used (e.g. vein graft or silicone/biodegradable materials).
- Source of non-vascularised nerve grafts includes medial and lateral antebrachial nerves of forearm, and sural nerve.

Postoperative considerations
- Mobilise as comfort allows. After day 3, range of motion exercises for joints that were not directly involved in the operation. Protect nerve repairs for 2/52, except for digital nerves.
- Patients should be informed of the long recovery time. Nerves grow at a rate of 1 mm/day once in the endoneurial tube (healing is affected by age of patient, mechanism, level and degree of injury, ischaemia, time to repair post injury).
- Non-sensate skin should be protected during this time.
- Referral to a hand therapist may be required for splinting and/or sensory re-education.

Additional considerations
Alternative treatments:
- No treatment
  - If neural regeneration cannot take place, a neuroma (benign tumour consisting of collagen-encased axon sprouts) will form. This may become painful if it is an area where it is subject to stimulation.[2] Absence of neural regeneration will also result in permanent loss of function or sensation in the affected distribution.
- Fibrin glue
  - There is controversy over the use of fibrin glue but some experimental studies suggest certain advantages over suture repair.[3] A clinical study using fibrin glue for brachial plexus injuries show a 30% decease in operative time and a slight slightly superior functional outcome compared to suture repair.[4] However there remain concerns regarding transmission of infection.
- Laser
  - This method is not in common use as there have been concerns regarding tensile strength and thermal effects of lasers.

CONSENT FORM
Name of procedure: Repair of peripheral nerve
Benefits:
 Return of function/sensation
Risks:
 General:
  Infection – no published figures available
  Bleeding
  Adverse scarring (including hypertrophic/keloid scars)
 Specific:
  Neuroma formation
  Persistence of symptoms
  Incomplete recovery (recovery is poorer with advancing age, more proximal
   injuries, crush/blast injuries, ischaemia, complete transection)
  Nerve grafting – donor scar and morbidity (numbness)
Procedure involves: General/regional/local anaesthesia

Key publications

Dvali L, Mackinnon S. The role of microsurgery in nerve repair and nerve grafting. *Hand Clin.* 2007; **23**(1)· 73–81 [5]

- This article reviews the role of microsurgery in nerve repair.
- Use of the operative microscope in this field has resulted in improved outcomes after peripheral nerve surgery.
- It has also allowed different types of nerve repair to be performed including techniques of nerve transfer and end-to-side repair.

References

1 Young L, Wray RC, Weeks PM. A randomized prospective comparison of fascicular and epineural digital nerve repairs. *Plast Reconstr Surg.* 1981; **68**(1): 89–92.
2 Dellon AL. Wound healing in nerve. *Clin Plast Surg.* 1990; **17**: 545.
3 Ornelas L, Padilla L, Di Silvio M, *et al.* Fibrin glue: an alternative technique for nerve coaptation: Part II, nerve regeneration and histomorphometric assessment. *J Reconstr Microsurg.* 2006; **22**(2): 123–8.
4 Narakas A. The use of fibrin glue in repair of peripheral nerves. *Orthop Clin North Am.* 1988; **19**(1): 187–99.
5 Dvali L, Mackinnon S. The role of microsurgery in nerve repair and nerve grafting. *Hand Clin.* 2007; **23**(1): 73–81.

Orthopaedic surgery

9.1 Compression hip screw for fractures of the femoral neck
Key points
For fixation of extracapsular neck of femur fractures, or undisplaced intracapsular femoral neck fractures.

Procedural considerations
- Preoperative investigations and a medical review if co-morbidities.
- There is a golden day to maximise the patient's fitness for surgery. Further delay increases the risk of bronchopneumonia, which is the principal cause of death after proximal femoral fracture.
- Mean length of stay is usually 1–2 weeks postoperatively – depends on patient, social and medical factors.
- Generaland/or regional anaesthesia (spinal/epidural) +/– nerve blocks (sciatic/femoral).
- The patient is placed supine on a traction table. A longitudinal incision is made on the lateral aspect of the upper thigh, starting at the level of the greater trochanter and directed distally. The proximal femur is exposed via this lateral approach. The dynamic hip screw system consists of a lag screw within a sliding barrel, allowing for 'dynamic' motion of the lag screw. The sliding barrel is part of a plate (usually 2- or 4-hole). The lag screw is inserted up the neck of the femur, ideally placed in the centre of the femoral neck (as seen on both an AP and lateral view using an image intensifier). The plate is attached to the side of the femur and held with screws.

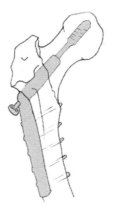

FIGURE 9.1 Dynamic hip screw fixation for hip fractures.

Postoperative considerations
- A drain may have been inserted for 24 hours.
- Further postoperative prophylactic antibiotics are usually given (depending on local policies).
- Routine bloods are performed 24–48 hours following surgery.
- Mobilise weight bearing as tolerated (unless otherwise indicated in the operation notes).
- A detailed social history and discharge plan should be formulated, as surgery is just the first part of the rehabilitation after this life-threatening injury.

Additional considerations
Non-surgical treatment should only be considered in non-ambulatory patients with multiple medical co-morbidities in whom the risk of surgery and anaesthesia would be very high.

CONSENT FORM
Name of procedure: Dynamic hip screw fixation proximal femur fracture (state which side)

Benefits:
Fixation of fracture allowing early weight bearing, mobilisation and decreased pain

Risks:[1,2]

General:
Confused state: 8%
Pressure sores: 6%
Chest infection: 5%
Urine retention: 4%
Deep vein thrombosis: 2%
Cardiac failure: 2.5%
Pulmonary embolus: 1%

Specific:
Overall complication rate in survivors is around 4%.
Mortality: (at 30 days): 8%; at 1 year, 15%–37%
Wound infection – superficial: 0.9%, deep: 0.9%
Lag screw cut out and failure of metalwork –detachment of plate from femoral shaft: 2%–5%
Non-union of fracture
Fracture displacement
Leg length discrepancy
Avascular necrosis of femoral head: 0.4%

Procedure involves: General anaesthesia and/or regional anaesthesia

---

Key publications
Chirodian N, Arch B, Parker MJ. Sliding hip screw fixation of trochanteric hip fractures: outcome of 1024 procedures. *Injury*. 2005; **36**: 793–800.[1]

- A prospective consecutive study of 1024 dynamic hip screw fixations in a single centre.

- Findings: 75% of fractures were classified unstable. Mortality rate at one year was 31%. Of the remaining 69% of patients, 95% had minimal or no pain. Overall complication rate was 3.6%. 2.6% of patients needed further surgery.
- Strengths: large numbers, prospective study, comprehensive demographic details of patients, good outcome measures and specific complications reviewed, no loss of patients to follow up, appropriate statistical analysis.

References
1 Chirodian N, Arch B, Parker MJ. Sliding hip screw fixation of trochanteric hip fractures: outcome of 1024 procedures. *Injury*. 2005; **36**: 793–800.
2 Hornby R, Grimley Evans J, Vardon V. Operative or conservative treatment for trochanteric fractures of the femur: a randomised epidemiological trial in elderly patients. *J Bone Joint Surg Br*. 1989; **71**(4): 619–23.

9.2 Hemiarthroplasty for intracapsular femoral fractures
Key points
Hemiarthroplasty is commonly done for displaced intracapsular fractures of the proximal femur (femoral neck) in elderly patients. With these fracture types, the blood supply to the femoral head is often compromised and therefore a replacement of the femoral head using a stemmed prosthesis is undertaken.

Procedural considerations
- Commonly done as an 'urgent' procedure following a neck of femur fracture. Current guidelines[1] recommend surgery should be performed within 48 hours of admission following injury, unless medical co-morbidities preclude this.
- Patients are often elderly and frail with multiple medical co-morbidities. They therefore require adequate preoperative work-up consisting of
  - up-to-date chest X-ray, ECG, screening blood tests, urine dipstick
  - adequate glycaemic control in diabetics
  - other investigations depending on mode of presentation and initial clinical findings.

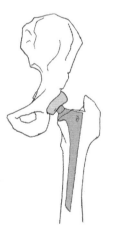

FIGURE 9.2 Hemiarthroplasty of the hip.

- Mean length of stay is usually 1–2 weeks postoperatively – depends on patient, social and medical factors.
- General or spinal anaesthetic.
- The patient is positioned in the lateral position with the affected side upwards.
  - An incision is made on the lateral aspect of the upper thigh and the hip joint is exposed through an antero-lateral approach.
  - The fractured femoral neck and head are retrieved and the remaining femoral neck is further cut to accept one of a number of prostheses types.
  - The medullary canal of the femur is prepared to accept either a cemented or uncemented hemiarthroplasty, which is then inserted.
  - The hemiarthroplasty is relocated into the native acetabulum, the soft tissues are repaired and the wound closed with either absorbable or non-absorbable material (including skin staples).

Postoperative considerations
- 3–4 perioperative doses of intravenous antibiotics are given, depending on local guidelines. The first is at induction of anaesthesia and the subsequent doses are within 24 hours of surgery.
- Mechanical and chemical thromboprophylaxis are given perioperatively until the patient's mobility obviates this need.
- Mobilise fully weight bearing as soon as they have recovered from the anaesthetic
- Postoperative blood tests include haemoglobin check as well as urea and electrolytes, typically performed on the first postoperative day.
- Careful attention should be paid to fluid balance postoperatively.
- Where non-absorbable suture material is used, this is usually removed at 10–14 days.
- Chest physiotherapy postoperatively to minimise risk of atelectasis and chest infection.

Additional considerations
Patients commonly drop down one level of mobility postop. compared with their pre-fracture status (e.g. if they were using one stick to mobilise, they may require two postop).[3]

CONSENT FORM
Name of procedure: Hemiarthroplasty of the hip (state which side)
Benefits:
> Treat fractured neck of femur
> Alleviate pain
> Improve functional outcome
Risks:[2,3]
> **General:**
> Infection: 1.2%
> Bleeding
> Adverse scarring
> Neurovascular damage
> Venous thromboembolism: 3% incidence of clinically relevant DVTs and 1% for clinically relevant pulmonary embolism[1]
> Anaesthetic complications

Specific:
  Dislocation: 1.7%
  Loosening: 0.8%
  Periprosthetic fracture: 1.2%
  Reduced mobility, mortality: 20%–33% at 1 year
Procedure involves: General and/or spinal anaesthesia

Key publications

Palmer SJ, Parker MJ, Hollingworth W. The cost and implications of reoperation after surgery for fracture of the hip. *J Bone Joint Surg Br.* 2000; **82**(6): 864–6.[2]

* Aims:
  – To determine the rate of complications, as well as financial and other implications of reoperation following different complications of hip fracture surgery.
* Methodology:
  – Prospective cohort study of hip fracture patients across two centres. Case note as well as clinical reviews to determine complication rates across different surgical treatment methods (sliding hip screw, cannulated screws, hemiarthroplasty), within a year of injury. Looked at rates of reoperation, length of hospital stay, mortality, infection, dislocation and peri-prosthetic fracture for hemiarthroplasties.
* Relevant findings:
  – 908 patients had a hemiarthroplasty for hip fracture; 1.2% had a deep infection requiring either surgical debridement or excision arthroplasty; 1.7% suffered a dislocation, all of whom were successfully relocated using closed methods; 0.8% suffered symptomatic loosening of the prosthesis requiring revision to a total hip arthroplasty; 1.2% patients had a fracture around the prosthesis.
* Strengths:
  – Large study population with prospectively collected data from more than one centre; clinically relevant outcome measures.
* Weakness:
  – Follow-up was limited to one year, which means later complications would be missed.

References

1 British Orthopaedic Association. *The Care of Patients with Fragility Fracture.* British Orthopaedic Association; 2007.
2 Palmer SJ, Parker MJ, Hollingworth W. The cost and implications of reoperation after surgery for fracture of the hip. *J Bone Joint Surg Br.* 2000; **82**(6): 864–6.
3 Parker MJ, Khan RJ, Crawford J, *et al.* Hemiarthroplasty versus internal fixation for displaced intracapsular hip fractures in the elderly: a randomised trial of 455 patients. *J Bone Joint Surg Br.* 2002; **84**(8): 1150–5.

9.3 Total hip replacement
Key points
Total hip replacement (THR) is commonly performed for osteoarthritis of the hip joint. Osteoarthritis is a degenerative joint disorder characterised by progressive loss of articular cartilage, new bone formation and capsular fibrosis.

Procedural considerations
- Preoperative assessments including up-to-date radiographs of hip joint (AP/lateral) +/– templating ball for preoperative templating.
- Length of stay usually 5–7 days – may be shorter or longer depending on patient, surgical and social factors.
- General or regional anaesthesia.
- A total hip replacement involves a surgical approach to the hip joint with the excision of the femoral head and preparation of the acetabulum (socket) and femoral shaft (stem). The prosthesis consists of a femoral stem, femoral head and acetabular component. Most modern prostheses are made of either a cobalt-chromium alloy or ceramic. The acetabular component is usually high-density polyethylene but may be metal or ceramic. The prosthesis can be either cemented in, or placed uncemented. Wound closure is usually with clips or sutures.

Postoperative considerations
- Patients may have a wound drain for 24 hours.
- Perioperative antibiotic prophylaxis is administered according to local guidelines.
- The patient will usually be on either a chemical or mechanical venous thromboprophylaxis regime or both.
- A check radiograph of the operated hip is taken postoperatively and prior to discharge.
- Full blood count, urea and electrolytes 24 hours following surgery.
- Mobilisation is usually full weight bearing and typically starts within 24–48 hours postoperatively.

Additional considerations
Alternative treatments:
- Non-operative treatment – analgesics, physiotherapy.

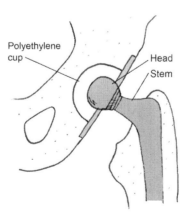

FIGURE 9.3 Total hip replacement.

- Operative therapy – hip resurfacing is another operative option. This involves surface replacement of the femoral head with preservation of most of the femoral neck and bone stock. This is relatively new technology and is not suitable for all patients in whom a THR is considered.

CONSENT FORM

Name of procedure: Primary total hip replacement (indicate which side)
Benefits:
> Relieve pain
> Improve mobility

Risks:[1]
General
> Infection (superficial and deep) – 1% risk of deep infection
> Venous thromboembolism: 40%
> Mortality: 1.3%

Specific
> Leg length discrepancy: 27%
> Dislocation: 3%
> Periprosthetic fracture
> Aseptic loosening
> Heterotopic ossification – abnormal bone formation within surrounding soft tissues: 15%–21%[2,3]
> Nerve injury: 1% – sciatic (79%), superior gluteal (17% direct lateral approach), femoral (13%), obturator (1.6%)[4,5,6]
> Limp and abductor weakness[7]

Procedure involves: General or regional anaesthesia

References

1 Northmore-Ball MD, Bannister GC, Mears DC, *et al. Clinical Challenges in Orthopaedics: the Hip*. London: Martin Dunitz; 2002. pp. 81–90.
2 De Lee J, Ferrari A, Charnley J. Ectopic bone formation following low-friction arthroplasty of the hip. *Clin Orthop*. 1976; **121**: 53–9.
3 Brooker AF, Bowerman JW, Robinson RA, *et al.* Ectopic ossification following total hip replacement: incidence and a method of classification. *J Bone Joint Surg Am*. 1973; **55**: 1629–32.
4 Schmalzried TP, Amstutz HC, Dorey FJ. Nerve palsy associated with total hip replacement: risk factors and prognosis. *J Bone Joint Surg Am*. 1991; **73**: 1074–80.
5 Weber ER, Daube JR, Coventry MB. Peripheral neuropathies associated with total hip arthroplasty. *J Bone Joint Surg Am*. 1976; **58**(1): 66–9.
6 Weale AE, Newman P, Ferguson IT, *et al.* Nerve injury after posterior and direct lateral approaches for hip replacement: a clinical and electrophysiological study. *J Bone Joint Surg Br*. 1996; **78**: 899–902.
7 Baker AS, Bitounis VC. Abductor function after total hip replacement: an electromyographic and clinical review. *J Bone Joint Surg Br*. 1989; **71**(1): 47–50.

9.4 Intramedullary nailing of a long bone
Key points
Intramedullary nailing is a method of fixation used for specific fracture types in long bones (femur, tibia, humerus). It can be used to treat both metaphyseal and diaphyseal fractures. The nail is inserted via an antegrade (proximal to distal) or retrograde (distal to proximal) approach.

The objective is to achieve a closed reduction of the fracture (i.e. without opening the fracture site itself) and pass the nail across the fracture whilst held reduced. Occasionally, the fracture site has to be opened to permit reduction. The nail is held with proximal and distal interlocking screws.

Procedural considerations
- Preoperative assessment.
- Intraoperative radiographic imaging is required.
- General or spinal anaesthesia.
- The procedure is carried out with the patient on a radiolucent table or traction table. Appropriate reduction manoeuvres (e.g. traction) may be performed and confirmed fluoroscopically prior to sterile preparation.
- A skin incision is made along the insertion point (proximal to the greater trochanter for antegrade femoral nails, anterior aspect of the knee for retrograde femoral or antegrade tibial nails). This is typically quite short (≤5 cm).
- An awl (coring device) or drill is used to create a cortical window at the insertion point and a guide wire is introduced into the medullary canal and passed across the fracture (with the fracture appropriately reduced).
- An appropriately sized nail is inserted over the guide wire with or without prior reaming of the medullary canal. This is held with interlocking screws distally and proximally. A femoral head screw may be used for femoral nails. The wound is closed with sutures and/or staples.

Postoperative considerations
- Perioperative antibiotic prophylaxis and thromboprophylaxis is undertaken according to local guidelines.

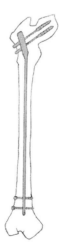

FIGURE 9.4 Intramedullary nailing.

- There is a significant risk of compartment syndrome following tibial fractures and more so following intramedullary nailing.[1] Close monitoring in the immediate postoperative period is mandatory.
- There is also a risk of fat embolism and respiratory compromise postoperatively.[2]
- Immediate weight bearing is usually encouraged depending on the quality of fixation (either partial or full weight bearing).
- Routine postoperative bloods should be taken to check haemoglobin levels, renal function and electrolytes, as well as other tests appropriate to the patient's co-morbidities.
- Initial follow up is typically at 2 weeks. Radiographs may be obtained at this stage.

Additional considerations
- Patients should be warned of the risk of anterior knee pain following the insertion of retrograde femoral or antegrade tibial nails.[3] This is particularly relevant in patients whose jobs involve a lot of kneeling as they may be unable to return to these jobs following surgery.

CONSENT FORM
Name of procedure: Intramedullary nailing (state bone and side)
Benefits:
    Treat fracture
    Promote bone healing
    Improve functional outcome
Risks:
  General:
    Infection: 1.8% for closed fractures[4]
    Bleeding
    Neurovascular damage
    Venous thromboembolism
    Fat embolism
    Anaesthetic complications
  Specific:
    Mal-union/non-union
    Compartment syndrome: 8%–12%[3]
    Anterior knee pain (tibial nails – up to 60% incidence[3])
    Metalwork failure
    Removal of metalwork
Procedure involves: General/regional anaesthesia

Key publications
Hooper GJ, Keddell RG, Penny ID. Conservative management or closed nailing for tibial shaft fractures: a randomised prospective trial. *J Bone Joint Surg Br.* 1991; **73**(1): 83–5.[5]
- Key message:
  - Intramedullary nailing is the most efficient method of treatment for closed displaced fractures of the tibial shaft.
- Study design:
  - Prospective randomised trial on matched groups of patients comparing conservative management (n=33) with intramedullary nailing (n=29) in closed or Grade I open tibial shaft fractures.

- – Conservative treatment consisted of a long leg cast for 4 weeks then conversion to a patellar-tendon-bearing cast, in which full weight bearing was allowed.
- – Patients treated by nailing were allowed to fully weight bear straight away.
- – Outcomes measures included time to union, non-union rates, incidence of mal-union and shortening, time in hospital, loss of joint movement (knee, ankle and subtalar joints) and incidence of complications (infection, nerve palsies, plaster sores, anterior knee pain).
- Findings:
  - – Shorter time to union in patients treated by intramedullary nailing (15.7 weeks vs. 18.3 weeks).
  - – Shorter time off work, fewer outpatient visits and radiographs in the group treated by intramedullary nailing.
  - – No non-unions in the nailed group (compared with one case in the conservatively treated group).
  - – Significantly more angular deformity and shortening in the conservatively treated group.
  - – Joint movements were regained earlier in the nailed group but similar in both groups by the end of treatment.
  - – Conservatively treated patients had no infections, three superficial nerve palsies, two cases of pressure sore and one re-fracture. Seven of the conservatively treated patients had failure of this method requiring subsequent surgical treatment.
  - – Patients treated by nailing had no episodes of infection, although there were three cases of transient wound problems. Six patients had problems with pain at the proximal end of the nail.
- Strengths:
  - – Prospective randomised study with matched groups.
  - – Stringent inclusion criteria.
  - – Clinically relevant outcome measures. Statistically significant findings.
- Weaknesses:
  - – Blinding not possible at time of assessment thus increasing the likelihood of observational/experimental bias.
  - – Single-centre study where intramedullary nailing was already the preferred treatment (possibility of experimenter bias – should be minimised by randomisation).
  - – No reference to type of nails used (reamed vs. unreamed) or whether they were statically or dynamically locked. These are all factors that have been subsequently shown to affect the measured outcomes.

References

1 Browner BD, Jupiter JB, Levine AM, *et al. Skeletal Trauma: basic science, management, reconstruction*. 3rd ed. Philadelphia, PA: WB Saunders; 2003. Ch. 57, pp. 2131–56, Tibial Shaft Fractures.
2 Christie J. The coagulative effects of fat embolisation during intramedullary manipulative procedures. *Tech Orthop*. 1996; **11**: 14–7.
3 Court-Brown CM, Will E, Christie J, *et al*. Reamed or unreamed nailing for closed tibial shaft fractures. *J Bone Joint Surg Br*. 1996; **78**(4): 580–83.
4 Court-Brown CM, Keating JF, McQueen MM. Infection after intramedullary nailing of the tibia: incidence and protocol for management. *J Bone Joint Surg Br*. 1992; **74**(5): 770–74.
5 Hooper GJ, Keddell RG, Penny ID. Conservative management or closed nailing for tibial shaft fractures: a randomised prospective trial. *J Bone Joint Surg Br*. 1991; **73**(1): 83–5.[5]

9.5 Diagnostic knee arthroscopy

Key points

The use of small incisions in the knee (minimally invasive technique) to provide portals through which arthroscopic instruments can be introduced, allowing visualisation of the knee joint as well as facilitating therapeutic procedures such as meniscectomy and removal of loose bodies. The most common portal sites are the anterolateral and antero-medial portals although more portals may be utilised.

Procedural considerations

- The patient may require preoperative radiographs and/or MRI of the affected knee to confirm the diagnosis prior to arthroscopy.
- Day case (unless there are specific patient-related or medical reasons requiring in-hospital stay).
- General anaesthetic although regional anaesthesia and even local anaesthetic can be used.
- The patient is placed supine on the operating table. A thigh tourniquet may be used. An examination under anaesthetic (EUA) is performed. An anterolateral portal is initially made in order to pass the endoscope into the knee joint. Then, depending on what other procedures are required, an anteromedial portal is made to allow other arthroscopic instruments to be introduced into the knee, under direct visualisation. During the procedure, digital photographs of the various compartments of the knee can be taken and stored. Local anaesthetic is often infiltrated into the incisions at the end of the operation to aid analgesia postoperatively. The incisions are either closed with sutures (usually just one will suffice per portal) or with steristrips. A bulky wool and crepe dressing applied and the tourniquet is then released.

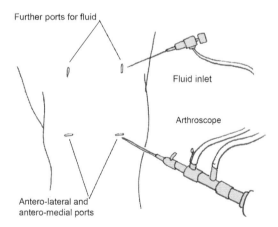

FIGURE 9.5 Portals used in arthroscopy. Note that the anterolateral and anteromedial portals are the most commonly deployed and are also referred to as inferolateral and inferomedial portals. Posterior portals are also sometimes used.

Postoperative considerations
- The bulky dressing is reduced to simple plasters or a slight circumferential dressing (e.g. tubigrip) within 24–48 hours.
- Mobilise fully weight bearing.

Additional considerations
- Knee arthroscopy can be done as a diagnostic and/or therapeutic procedure.
- It may also be done as an adjunct to a knee washout for sepsis.

CONSENT FORM
Name of procedure: Examination under anaesthesia and knee arthroscopy (indicate side) +/– proceed (important as other procedures may be necessary intraoperatively)

Benefits:
    Diagnosis and potential treatment of knee symptoms
    Obtain tissue samples
    Eradicate infection (depending on the indication for arthroscopy)

Risks:[1]

General:
    Pain – intra-articular local anaesthetic can reduce this problem.
    Thromboembolism: 0.1%–7%. (No indication as yet that routine thromboprophylaxis is needed in arthroscopic surgery. Minimising tourniquet and operating times and early mobilisation reduce this risk.)
    Infection: 0.08%–0.42%

Specific:
    Haemarthrosis: 1%
    Effusion and synovitis – up to 15% risk of an effusion, which may be prolonged.
    Synovial fistula – rare
    Temporary paresis due to tourniquet use. Prolonged tourniquet times (over 60 minutes) are associated with an increased risk of complications.
    Compartment syndrome – case reports of it occurring as a result of a defect in the capsule.
    Intra-articular damage from the arthroscopic instruments – potential sites of injury include the anterior meniscal horns and the articular cartilage.
    Complex regional pain syndrome – an uncommon complication resulting in pain and skin/soft tissue changes around the knee. Its aetiology is poorly understood.
    Neurological injury – as a result of direct trauma, compartment syndrome or tourniquet use – rare (0.01%–0.06%), saphenous nerve is most commonly injured.
    Vascular injury – very rare. More likely with therapeutic arthroscopy involving powered instruments. Injury to the popliteal artery can lead to amputation. Injury to the superior lateral geniculate artery can occur during a lateral release and may result in a haemarthrosis.

Procedure involves: General/regional/local anaesthesia

Reference
1 Allum R. Complications of arthroscopy of the knee. *J Bone Joint Surg Br*. 2002; **84**(7): 937–45.

9.6 Total knee replacement

Key points

Total knee arthroplasty – or total knee replacement (TKR) – is a procedure commonly performed for destructive arthritis of the knee joint. It involves removal of the destroyed articular cartilage, fixation of metal components to the femur and tibia and interposition of a polyethylene liner between these to create a new weight-bearing surface.

Procedural considerations

- Up-to-date radiographs should be obtained (no older than 6 months). These typically include a standing antero-posterior, lateral and skyline patellofemoral views of the knee. Some surgeons obtain long-leg alignment radiographs (hip to ankle) of both legs.
- Length of stay is typically 5 days in uncomplicated cases.
- TKR can be done under general or regional anaesthesia.
- With the patient supine on the operating table, a thigh tourniquet is applied. Sterile preparation is applied from the mid thigh to the foot.
- The tourniquet is inflated and a skin incision is made over the anterior aspect of the knee, extending from the distal thigh, over the medial third of the patella, to just medial to the tibial tubercle. The knee is then entered usually through a medial para-patellar approach.
- The distal femur and proximal tibia are resected using a system of cutting blocks and guides such that the resulting surfaces are fashioned to accept the prostheses. The tibial and femoral components are cemented onto the prepared surfaces.
- The patellar articular surface may also be resected and replaced with a plastic button although this is not always done.[1]
- A polyethylene insert is placed on the tibial component, the knee is reduced, washed out and closed, often over a drain (which may be an autologous re-transfusion drain).

Postoperative considerations

- A bulky dressing is usually applied for the first 24–48 hours, after which it is reduced to allow mobilisation of the knee.

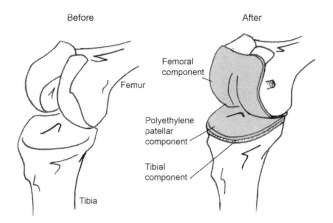

FIGURE 9.6 Total knee replacement.

- If an autologous re-transfusion drain is used, it is common practice to open the drain 20 minutes after the tourniquet is released.
- Autologous blood may be given for up to 12 hours postop. after which most manufacturers recommend discarding collected blood. Drains are usually taken out at 24 hours postop.
- A haemoglobin check should be undertaken at 24–48 hours postop. along with renal function tests and other blood tests if indicated.
- Early mobilisation of the knee is the goal, usually within 24 hours, and the patient is allowed to fully weight bear unless otherwise stated in the postoperative instructions.
- Non-absorbable skin closure material is taken out at 10–14 days postoperatively.

Additional considerations
- TKR is done as a quality-of-life modifying procedure to alleviate pain and improve mobility.
- Alternatives to this treatment include non-operative measures such as analgesics (oral and transdermal), activity modification and the use of mobility aids.
- Other surgical alternatives include 'partial arthroplasties' such as patello-femoral arthroplasty and unicompartmental knee replacements, but these are only successful in carefully selected patients and may ultimately require revision to a total knee replacement.[2,3]
- Osteotomies around the knee can also be performed, usually as a temporary measure in the younger patient, to off-load affected compartments in the knee. The goal of this is usually to slow disease progression and buy time until arthroplasty becomes necessary. However, there is no definitive evidence of its efficacy over conservative treatment.[4]

CONSENT FORM
Name of procedure: Total knee replacement (indicate which side)
Benefits:
       Alleviate pain
       Improve mobility
       Correct deformity
Risks:[5,6]
  General:
       Infection: <1% for deep infections
       Impaired wound healing: 5%–10%. (Of these, 10% develop wound infections if not treated expeditiously.)
       Bleeding
       Neurovascular damage
       Venous thromboembolism: 2.4% – incidence of subclinical below-knee DVTs thought to be much higher (>50%[7])
       Anaesthetic complications (myocardial infarction, pneumonia)
       Mortality: 0.4% at 1 month and 1.8% at 1 year
  Specific:
       Persistent or recurrent symptoms
       Stiffness possibly requiring further manipulation
       Swelling
       Loosening

Periprosthetic fracture
Extensor mechanism disruption
Complication requiring revision: 5.6% at an average of 6 years
Complication requiring amputation: 0.12%
Procedure involves: General/regional anaesthesia

Key publications
Roberts VI, Esler CN, Harper WMA. 15-year follow-up study of 4606 primary total knee replacements. *J Bone Joint Surg Br.* 2007; **89**(11): 1452–6.[6]

- Aims:
  - To determine the long-term outcomes following total knee arthroplasty in terms of patient and implant survival, patient satisfaction, pain and quality of life.
  - To analyse the impact of different variables on the aforementioned outcomes.
- Methodology:
  - Observational study of all primary TKRs performed in one healthcare region from 1990–1992.
  - Prospectively collected data from Regional Joint Registry (patient demographics, medical, operative and implant details).
  - Patient-administered questionnaire enquiring about satisfaction, presence of pain, quality of life – on a visual analog scale (VAS) – and revision procedures.
  - Revisions were identified using the revision arthroplasty database.
- Results:
  - 4606 TKRs in 4390 patients, 64% females, mean age 70 yrs.
  - Mortality: 0.4% 1-month mortality, 1.8% 1-year mortality – 47% of patients alive at 15 years.
  - Cumulative implant survival of 97.5% at 5 yrs, 94.4% at 10 yrs and 92.2% at 15 yrs.
  - 5.6% revision rate at an average of 76 months (range 1–185 months).
  - 85% satisfaction rate amongst respondents to questionnaire.
  - Patient satisfaction not affected by age at primary surgery. However, males, patients with OA as primary diagnosis, and patients requiring revision were more likely to be dissatisfied.
  - Older patients, females, and those with the primary prosthesis still in situ, experienced pain less often.
  - Average VAS of 58.9 for quality of life (scale of 0–100, 100 being 'best' score). Not affected by any of the observed variables.
- Strengths:
  - Multicentre, multisurgeon series.
  - Large patient numbers.
  - Prospectively collected data.
  - Clinically relevant outcome measures with patient-focused outcomes.
- Weaknesses:
  - 10% loss to follow up.
  - 58% response rate to questionnaires with the possibility of responder bias.

References
1 Meneghini RM. Should the patella be resurfaced in primary total knee arthroplasty? an evidence-based analysis. *J Arthroplasty.* 2008; **23**(7 Suppl.): 11–14.
2 McAllister CM. The role of unicompartmental knee arthroplasty versus total knee

arthroplasty in providing maximal performance and satisfaction. *J Knee Surg*. 2008; **21**(4): 286–92.

3 Leadbetter WB. Patellofemoral arthroplasty in the treatment of patellofemoral arthritis: rationale and outcomes in younger patients. *Orthop Clin North Am*. 2008; **39**(3): 363–80.

4 Brouwer RW, Raaij van TM, Bierma-Zeinstra SM, *et al*. Osteotomy for treating knee osteoarthritis Cochrane Database Syst Rev. 2007; 3: CD004019.

5 NIH. Consensus Statement on total knee replacement. *NIH Consens State Sci Statements*. 2003; **20**(1): 1–34.

6 Roberts VI, Esler CN, Harper WM. A 15-year follow-up study of 4606 primary total knee replacements. *J Bone Joint Surg Br*. 2007; **89**(11): 1452–6.

7 Warwick D, Harrison J, Whitehouse S, *et al*. A randomised comparison of a foot pump and low-molecular-weight heparin in the prevention of deep-vein thrombosis after total knee replacement. *J Bone Joint Surg Br*. 2002; **84**(3): 344–50.

9.7 Application of an external fixator

Key points

An external fixator is used to stabilise a fracture without violating the zone of injury. It involves the placement of pins in the bone proximal and distal to the fracture site and fixing these to an external system of rods and connectors, such that little movement is permitted at the fracture site whilst it heals. This permits fracture fixation with minimal disruption to the soft tissues around the fracture. In open fractures, soft tissue reconstruction may be required. The patient should be warned of this and pins should be placed to facilitate subsequent procedures.

Procedural considerations

- Preoperative assessments including radiographs showing the full length of the bone (including the joints above and below).
- Intraoperative radiographic imaging is required.[2]
- General anaesthesia although regional techniques may be used.[2]
- Treatment of other aspects of the injury may be necessary at the same time (e.g. irrigation and debridement, with soft-tissue coverage for open fractures).
- After appropriate positioning and sterile preparation, partially threaded pins are inserted via percutaneous stab incisions into the proximal and distal bone segments away from the fracture site. This is done under image guidance to ensure bicortical hold of the pins.
- The pins are then connected via a system of rods and connectors. These are adjusted

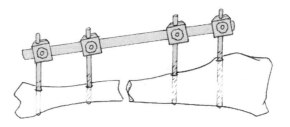

FIGURE 9.7 External fixator applied to the tibia. Note that the pins are placed away from the fracture site.

to ensure satisfactory fracture reduction and alignment and the connectors are tightened to provide a semi-rigid construct.
- The pin sites are dressed, usually with non-adhesive material.

Postoperative considerations
- Perioperative antibiotic prophylaxis and thromboprophylaxis according to local guidelines.
- Elevation of the limb may be desirable to reduce dependent oedema (caution in cases of vascular compromise).[2]
- Length of stay in hospital will depend on injury type and associated injuries. Early mobilisation is encouraged, non-weight bearing or partial weight bearing, depending on injury and quality of fixation.
- Pin sites should be inspected, cleaned and re-dressed regularly to minimise risk of loosening and infection. This responsibility will often be shared with the patient and appropriate education is vital to success.
- Repeat radiographs of the full length of the involved bone should be performed at 48 hours to check for further displacement.
- The connectors may need to be further tightened at 48–72 hours (on the ward).
- Early mobilisation of joints around the fracture site is essential to prevent the development of contractures.[1,2]
- The patient will need to be followed up in the outpatients' clinic at regular intervals with radiographs to ensure maintenance of reduction and assess degree of bone healing.

Additional considerations
- An external fixator may be used as a temporary fixation device or as definitive fixation for a fracture.
- If used as the definitive mode of treatment, the patient should be counselled as to the duration of use and its implications for function (a minimum of 6 weeks is typical, often up to 5 months in the lower limb to allow adequate bone healing[1,2]).
- Although the commonest use is in the trauma situation, there are other applications of external fixators including limb-deformity correction, management of non-unions, limb-lengthening procedures and arthrodesis.
- The fixator will have to be removed after adequate healing is achieved, usually requiring a second anaesthetic.

CONSENT FORM
Name of procedure: Application of external fixator (state side and bone)
Benefits:
> Promote fracture healing
> Preserve soft tissues around fracture
> Restore function
Risks:[3]
> **General:**
>> Infection
>> Bleeding
>> Neurovascular damage
>> Venous thromboembolism
>> Anaesthetic complications

Specific:
Mal-union
Delayed union
Non-union
Contractures
Compartment syndrome
Further surgery (removal of metalwork)
Procedure involves: General/regional anaesthesia

Key publications

Lethaby A, Temple J, Santy J. Pin site care for preventing infections associated with external bone fixators and pins. Cochrane Database Syst Rev. 2008; 4: CD004551.[4]

- Aim:
  - To investigate the effect of cleansing solutions, dressing types and frequency of pin-site care on the rate of pin-site infection following the use of percutaneous pins as part of an external fixator or skeletal traction system.
- Methodology:
  - A systematic review of randomised controlled trials. Trials were selected based on pre-defined criteria.
- Results:
  - Six randomised controlled trials met the inclusion criteria with a total of 349 participants.
  - Three trials compared cleansing regimens with no cleansing, two trials compared different cleansing solutions and one trial compared daily vs. weekly cleansing using the same solution and dressings.
  - Four trials compared dressings.
  - One trial reported lower infection rates (9%) when cleansing was done with half-strength hydrogen peroxide and Xeroform dressings were applied, as compared with >26% infection rates with other regimens. However, this may have been a chance difference.
  - None of the other trials identified a difference in infection rates between comparison groups.
- Conclusions:
  - There is insufficient evidence in the literature to affirm superiority of any pin-care regimen for minimising risk of infection.
  - Adequately powered randomised controlled trials are required to investigate effect of pin-care regimen on infection rates.
  - Studies must factor in extraneous factors such as antibiotic usage and the use of pre-drilling at the time of infection, which may have an effect on the measured outcome.

References

1 Bucholz RW, Heckman JD, Court-Brown C, *et al*. Principles of external fixation. In: *Rockwood and Green's Fractures in Adults*. 6th ed. Philadelphia, PA: Lippincott Williams & Wilkins; 2006.
2 Sisk TD. General principles and techniques of external fixation. *Clin Orthop*. 1983; **180**: 96–100.
3 Green SA. Complications of external skeletal fixation. *Clin Orthop*. 1983; **180**: 109–16.

4 Lethaby A, Temple J, Santy J. Pin site care for preventing infections associated with external bone fixators and pins. Cochrane Database Syst Rev. 2008; 4: CD004551.

9.8 Operative fixation of ankle fractures
Key points
Reduction and internal fixation is indicated for open fractures, and closed fractures which are unstable with significant talar shift (displaced bi- or tri-malleolar fractures, fracture-dislocation of ankle joint). This usually entails using a one-third tubular plate and screws over the lateral malleolus and screws to fix the medial malleolus. A syndesmotic screw may also be needed if there is evidence of a syndesmotic injury.

Procedural considerations
- If the ankle is displaced in the emergency department, it should be reduced immediately before X-ray to protect the skin and prevent synovial fistula.
- Routine preoperative preparation. Be aware of patients who are diabetic and/or on warfarin.
- Length of stay is dependent on how much swelling is present around the ankle at the time of presentation. If there is gross swelling, operative fixation will be delayed until such time as the swelling has decreased sufficiently to enable adequate closure of the soft tissues following operative fixation. The old adage 'from 6 hours to 6 days' may apply. During the patient's inpatient stay, strict elevation of the leg and use of ice packs to reduce the swelling is advised.
- General/regional anaesthesia.
- A lateral incision is made, centred over the lateral malleolus, and the fracture identified and reduced. A 1/3 tubular plate of the appropriate length is applied onto the fibula and held with screws. If there has been a medial malleolus fracture also, this may be fixed using a medial incision and partially threaded screws. Alternatively, a tension band wire technique may be employed. At this stage, the syndesmosis is assessed and if damaged, a syndesmotic screw can be used. The fixation is performed with the aid of an image intensifier.

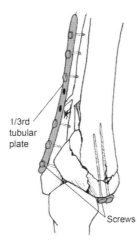

1/3rd tubular plate

Screws

FIGURE 9.8 Operative fixation of ankle fracture.

Postoperative considerations
- A below-knee plaster of Paris backslab is usually applied and the patient's leg is elevated.
- Non-weight bearing for a period of up to 6 weeks.
- Any sutures or clips used to close the skin will be removed at 2 weeks postoperatively and a wound check performed in clinic.

Additional considerations
- Non-operative treatment in a below-knee plaster could be used, as long as satisfactory anatomical reduction of the ankle joint has been achieved with closed reduction techniques. This will require close observation in the outpatient setting for the first 1–2 weeks post injury, with repeat X-ray checks to ensure that the fracture has not displaced within the plaster. The patient will need to be mobilised non-weight bearing for up to 6 weeks. Non-operative treatment may be appropriate if the patient is very elderly with multiple medical co-morbidities, which would significantly increase the risks of surgery and anaesthesia.

CONSENT FORM

Name of procedure: Open reduction and internal fixation of ankle (state which side)

Benefits:
> Anatomical reduction of ankle joint
> Early ankle motion preventing stiffness
> Improve functional outcome from injury

Risks:
> **General:**
>> Stiffness
>> Infection/wound complications: 1.4%–4%[1,2,3]
>> Venous thromboembolism – pulmonary embolism: 0.34%[3], DVT: 3.5%[5]
>> Death: 1%[3]

> **Specific:**
>> Loss of fixation
>> Posttraumatic arthritis: up to 14%[1]
>> Non-union/mal-union
>> Hardware prominence and failure[3]
>> Pain
>> Nerve injury (saphenous and posterior tibial medially, superficial peroneal and sural laterally)
>> Vascular injury (saphenous vein)
>> Late pain/complex regional pain syndrome: 31%[4]
>> Hardware prominence and failure: 23%[4]
>> Need for below-knee amputation: 0.2%[3]
>> Need for revision surgery: 0.8%[3]
>> Patients with poorly controlled diabetes and/or peripheral vascular disease have significantly higher complications rates of infection (7%) and need for below-knee amputation: 3%[3]

Procedure involves: General and/or regional anaesthesia

References
1 Lindsjo U. Operative treatment of ankle fracture dislocations: a follow up study of 306/321 consecutive cases. *Clin Orthop*. 1985; **199**: 28–38.
2 Phillips WA, Schwartz HS, Keller CS, *et al.* A prospective randomised study of the management of severe ankle fractures. *J Bone Joint Surg Am*. 1985; **67**: 67–78.
3 SooHoo NF, Krenek L, Eagan MJ, *et al.* Complication rates following open reduction and internal fixation of ankle fractures. *J Bone Joint Surg Am*. 2009; **91**: 1042–9.
4 Brown OL, Dirschl DR, Obremskey WT. Incidence of hardware-related pain and its effect on functional outcomes after open reduction and internal fixation of ankle fractures. *J Orthop Trauma*. 2001; **15**: 271–4.
5 Leyes M, Torres R, Guillén P. Complications of open reduction and internal fixation of ankle fractures. *Foot Ankle Clin*. 2003; **8**(1): 131–47.

9.9 Lumbar discectomy
Key points
Surgical removal of all or part of a lumbar vertebral disc which has prolapsed, causing mechanical nerve root compression and/or chemical irritation, leading to subsequent leg pain (sciatica).

A discectomy may be performed as a microdiscectomy (using a microscope) or as an open/mini-open procedure. Both approaches have similar outcomes.

Procedural considerations
- MRI lumbar spine, plain radiographs lumbar spine (standing AP/lateral).
- Need to stop warfarin, aspirin, clopidogrel preoperatively.
- Length of stay: 1–2 days.
- General anaesthesia.
- Patient is placed prone on a spinal operating table. A small midline incision is made over the lumbar spine, centred over the level of the disc protrusion. An image intensifier is used to confirm the position of the disc.

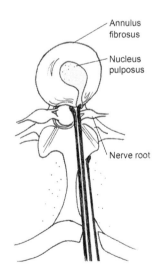

Annulus fibrosus

Nucleus pulposus

Nerve root

FIGURE 9.9 Lumbar discectomy.

Postoperative considerations

- Mobilise postoperatively as comfort allows. If a drain is present, this is removed at 24 hours postoperatively. The wound should be checked prior to discharge to ensure that there has been no CSF leak. The presence of a profound positional headache associated with a clear wound discharge, should alert the surgeon to a potential iatrogenic dural tear.

Additional considerations

- The majority of patients (75%) who present for the first time with symptoms of sciatica get better within 1 month or so. The mainstay of treatment initially is therefore adequate and appropriate analgesia (especially NSAIDs) and early mobilisation. Physiotherapy is also included in the non-operative treatment of herniated discs. Nerve root injections (using a combination of local anaesthetic and steroid) may also be performed under radiological guidance.
- There is no clear evidence that surgery has any positive or negative effect on the natural history of disc disease and at 2 years, patients who had surgery and those who did not, had similar improvements in symptoms.

CONSENT FORM

Name of procedure: Lumbar discectomy (state level and side)/micro or open discectomy

Benefits:
  Improve leg pain symptoms
  Quicker recovery[5]
  May improve back pain
  Pre-existing numbness or weakness in the legs may still persist despite surgery.

Risks:[1,2,3,4]

  General:
    Death: <1 in 0.14% – a fatal pulmonary embolus or catastrophic haemorrhage.
    Infection: 0%–4% – usually superficial but in <1% cases, there is deep infection which requires further surgery (washout of wound) plus prolonged intravenous antibiotics. There is a higher risk of infection in patients with diabetes, or who are immunocompromised, or have been on steroids.

  Specific:[3,4]
    Pyogenic discitis: 2%, epidural abscess: 0.3%
    Paralysis: <0.33% – secondary to an extradural spinal haematoma (especially if the patient has been on warfarin or has a bleeding disorder) or iatrogenic durotomy causing a CSF leak. May be as a result of damage to the vascular supply to the spinal cord or nerves causing a cord infarct.
    Iatrogenic durotomy (dural tear): 3%–5% of primary discectomies. Higher risk in revision surgery or if there has been previous surgery at the operative site (as a result of scarring). If there has been a durotomy, this can be repaired intraoperatively by using a fat patch or using sutures. A drain (but not under vacuum suction) may be inserted to allow free drainage of any CSF. Dural tears may lead to positional headaches, meningitis, wound complications and pseudomeningocoele formation. The patient will need to lie flat for 24 hours and may require IV fluids.

Spinal nerve damage – either iatrogenic or as a result of scarring from the prolapsed disc. Stretching (neuropraxia) of the nerve may occur as a result of pushing the nerve to one side in order to remove the underlying disc. Rarely, damage to the blood supply of the nerve can cause the nerve to infarct.

Damage to blood vessels – rare: 0.1%, but can be fatal (aorta damaged) or lead to limb loss as a result of damage to a major artery to the legs.

Wrong level – the wrong disc or site. Intraoperative fluoroscopy is routinely performed to minimise the risk of this happening.

Failure to improve symptoms: 5%

Worsening pain symptoms: 1%

Recurrence of disc prolapse – either at the same level or levels above or below: 3%–19%

Urinary retention – more common with advancing age and if patients are on beta-blockers preoperatively

Instability

Procedure involves: General anaesthesia

Key publications

Morgan-Hough CVJ, Jones PW, Eisenstein SM. Primary and revision lumbar discectomy: a 16-year review from one centre. *J Bone Joint Surg Br.* 2003; **85**(6): 871–4.[3]

● Summary:
  – Retrospective review of 553 patients who underwent primary discectomy from a single centre and single surgeon series. Revision rate of 7.9%. Complication rate of 8.7%.
● Strengths:
  – Large numbers, standard operative procedure, follow-up 1 year to 16 years, appropriate statistics, low numbers of loss to follow-up (4)
● Weaknesses:
  – Retrospective review, single surgeon series and single centre.

References

1 Weinstein JN, Tosteson TD, Lurie JD, *et al.* Surgical vs. non-operative treatment for lumbar disk herniation: the Spine Patient Outcomes Research Trial (SPORT): a randomized trial. *JAMA.* 2006; **296**(20): 2441–50.
2 Gibson JN, Waddell G. Surgical interventions for lumbar disc prolapse. Cochrane Database Syst Rev. 2007; 1: CD001350.
3 Morgan-Hough CVJ, Jones PW, Eisenstein SM. Primary and revision lumbar discectomy: a 16-year review from one centre. *J Bone Joint Surg Br.* 2003; **85**(6): 871–4.
4 Tafazal SI, Sell PJ. Incidental durotomy in lumbar spine surgery: incidence and management. *Eur Spine J.* 2005; **14**(3): 287–90.
5 Weber H. The natural history of disc herniation and the influence of intervention. *Spine.* 1994; **19**(19): 2234–8.

10

Urology

10.1 Cystourethroscopy
Key points
Cystourethroscopy is an endoscopic examination of the urethra and bladder.

Indicated for the investigation of haematuria and irritative lower urinary tract symptoms, biopsy and diathermy to lesions, insertion and removal of stents, removal of stones and follow up of patients with previous bladder carcinoma.[1]

Procedural considerations
- Pre-procedure – blood tests to assess renal function.
- Assessment of risk factors for bleeding, e.g. aspirin, warfarin.
- Day-case procedure.
- A recent review concludes no need for prophylactic antibiotics (but only low to moderate evidence).[2]
- Cystoscope may be flexible or rigid. Flexible cystoscopy is usually done under local anaesthetic, whereas rigid cystoscopy requires a general anaesthetic.
- Local anaesthesia (2% lignocaine gel), however, recent evidence does not show significant reduction in pain in men undergoing flexible cystoscopy with the use of lignocaine gel.[3]

Postoperative considerations
- Depending on indication for procedure a catheter may be inserted at conclusion.
- Patient must pass urine before being discharged.

CONSENT FORM
Name of procedure: Cystourethroscopy +/– biopsy +/– insertion/removal of stents +/– removal of stones
Benefits:
    Examination of lower urinary tract and bladder
Risks:
  General:
    Discomfort
  Specific:
    Bleeding – post-procedure mild haematuria is common
    Urinary tract infection – uncommon
    Urethral stricture – very rare
    Urinary retention – uncommon
    Epididymitis – rare[4]
    Perforation – very rare
Procedure involves: Local/general anaesthesia

References

1 Reynard J, Brewster S, Biers S. *Oxford Handbook of Urology*. Oxford: Oxford University Press; 2005.
2 Laguna Pes MP, Geerlings SE, Goossens A. Antibiotic prophylaxis in urologic procedures: a systematic review. *Eur Urol*. 2008; **54**(6): 1270–86.
3 Patel AR, Jones JS, Babineau D. Lidocaine 2% gel versus plain lubricating gel for pain reduction during flexible cystoscopy: a meta-analysis of prospective, randomized, controlled trials. *J Urol*. 2008; **179**(3): 986–90.
4 Gaynes SM. *Cystoscopy*. Available at: www.emedicinehealth.com/cystoscopy/page10_em.htm (accessed 13 June 2010).

10.2 Operative treatment of testicular torsion

Key points

Testicular torsion is a surgical emergency where arterial inflow to, and venous outflow from, the testicle is impeded due to the spermatic cord becoming twisted on its axis. The testis is therefore at risk of ischaemia and infarction. For prepubertal and adolescent boys, exploration is performed with attempted salvage of the ipsilateral testis. If torsion is confirmed, contralateral orchidopexy is recommended. The recommendations for neonates with an acute scrotum remain controversial, due to the low testicular salvage rate and low contralateral incidence of torsion.

Procedural considerations

- Pre-procedure – all efforts should be focused on arranging for surgical exploration as soon as possible. Surgery should not be delayed by performing imaging studies and/or laboratory studies.
- General anaesthesia.
- Paramedian, transverse or midline scrotal incision. If the diagnosis of torsion is confirmed, the testicle is detorsioned and the viability assessed. An orchidectomy (if not viable) or orchidopexy (if viable) is performed. A contralateral orchidopexy is also performed as the testicular deformity (bell clapper) predisposing to torsion, is generally bilateral. The tunica vaginalis is everted and a few sutures are passed through the dartos and tunica albuginea.

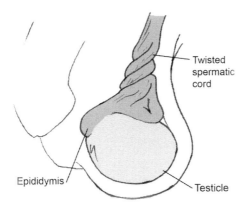

FIGURE 10.1 Testicular torsion.

Postoperative considerations
- Mobilise as comfortable.

Additional considerations
Alternative treatments:
- No treatment – this will lead to loss of testis. Rates of 55%–80% of testicular loss have been reported, mainly due to delay in treatment.[1,2]
- Medical therapy – manual untwisting using the 'open book' method can immediately relieve symptoms. However, this is a difficult procedure (thus not often performed), is only a temporary measure until definitive surgery can be performed, and does not obviate the need for surgery – 100% testicular salvage rates have been reported, converting an acute emergency into an urgent or elective case.[3]

CONSENT FORM

Name of procedure: Testicular exploration +/– salvage and orchidopexy
Benefits:
    Salvage of testicle
    Prevention of recurrent torsion
Risks:
    General:
        Infection – abscess formation in 30% of testes in animal models, with use of non-absorbable sutures[6]
        Bleeding/haematoma
        Adverse scarring
    Specific:
        Testicular atrophy – directly related to time elapsed since onset of symptoms, in adolescents.
            If surgery performed within 4–6 hours: salvage rates approximately 90%. At 12 hours 50%, after 24 hours 10%[4]
            Perinatal – <5% salvage rate
        Recurrence
            Rare but may occur many years later[5]
            There is a higher incidence of recurrent torsion after fixation using absorbable sutures.[6]
            Lower rate of adhesion formation and thus recurrence with eversion of tunica vaginalis during fixation.[6]
        Impaired testicular function/subfertility
            Significant subfertility exists in patients following unilateral testicular torsion, implying bilateral testicular disease. Experimental data suggesting a possible ischaemia-reperfusion injury damaging the blood-testes barrier. Evidence in humans is sparse.[7]
Procedure involves: General anaesthesia

Key publications
Tryfonas G, Violaki A, Tsikopoulos G, *et al.* Late postoperative results in males treated for testicular torsion during childhood. *J Pediatr Surg.* 1994; **29**(4): 553–6.[8]
- Retrospective review of 75 patients who were treated for testicular torsion.
- Operative detorsion with bilateral orchidopexy in 64 cases.

- Orchidectomies performed in 11 cases.
- 25 patients were re-examined 1 to 12 years after the surgery.
- Testicular atrophy correlated with duration of symptoms and operative finding.
- If torsion lasted more than 24 hours and viability of the testis was questionable, subsequent atrophy resulted.

References

1 Chapman RH, Walton AJ. Torsion of the testis and its appendages. *Br Med J.* 1972; **1**(5793): 164–6.
2 Bennett S, Nicholson MS, Little TM. Torsion of the testis: why is the prognosis so poor? *Br Med J (Clin Res Ed).* 1987; **294**: 824.
3 Cattolica EV. Preoperative manual detorsion of the torsed spermatic cord. *J Urol.* 1985; **133**(5): 803–5.
4 Davenport M, ABC of general surgery in children: acute problems of the scrotum. *BMJ.* 1996; **312**: 435–7.
5 Mor Y, Pinthus JH, Nadu A, *et al.* Testicular fixation following torsion of the spermatic cord: does it guarantee prevention of recurrent torsion events? *J Urol.* 2006; **175**(1): 171–3.
6 Sells H, Moretti KL, Burfield GD. Recurrent torsion after previous testicular fixation. *ANZ J Surg.* 2002; **72**(1): 46–8.
7 Koşar A, Küpeli B, Alçigir G, *et al.* Immunologic aspect of testicular torsion: detection of antisperm antibodies in contralateral testicle. *Eur Urol.* 1999; **36**(6): 640–4.
8 Tryfonas G, Violaki A, Tsikopoulos G, *et al.* Late postoperative results in males treated for testicular torsion during childhood. *J Pediatr Surg.* 1994; **29**(4): 553–6.

10.3 Male sterilisation: vasectomy
Key points

This is a form of male contraception. It involves an operation to occlude the vas deferens bilaterally with the intention of permanent birth control. A vasectomy does not affect sex drive, erectile function, or ejaculation. The semen, however, will not contain sperm. The procedure should be considered permanent but in certain cases can be reversed although with no guarantee that fertility will be restored.

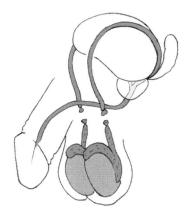

FIGURE 10.2 Vasectomy.

Procedural considerations
- Day-case under LA (GA is also an option).
- 10–15 minutes.
- Conventional vasectomy: either one midline or two small scrotal skin incisions are made in the scrotum and each vas deferens is pulled out, cut, and a small section removed. The ends of the vas deferens are then tied or diathermied and replaced. The skin incisions are then closed with sutures or steristrips.
- 'No scalpel' method: a sharp haemostat is used to open the skin at a single point rather than with a scalpel. This method uses a vasal nerve block which is thought to provide better anaesthesia.[1,2]
- 'Vas-Clip' method: this method clips the vas deferens instead of cutting it.

Postoperative considerations
- Simple analgesia for tender scrotum for a few days.
- Supportive and disposable underwear for a few days.
- Return to work within 2 days usually.
- No heavy lifting or strenuous exercise for 1 week.
- Contraceptive effects are not immediate because viable sperm must be cleared form the vas deferens. Therefore, alternative methods of contraception must be used until semen is clear of sperm.
- Semen test after 8 weeks and retested several weeks later if there is sperm in the semen.
- Continued testing until semen is clear of sperm.

Additional considerations
- The commonest requests for reversal are remarriage after divorce or after the death of a partner, the death of a child, a desire for more children, or psychological problems related to the vasectomy.[3]
- The total failure rate of condoms is approximately 1%.[4]

CONSENT FORM
Name of procedure: Male sterilisation/vasectomy
Benefits:
   Permanent contraception
Risks:
   General:
   Bleeding: 2% with conventional and 0.1% with no-scalpel method[2,5]
   Infection: 3.5% with conventional and 0.9% with no-scalpel method[2,5]
   Specific:
   Irreversible
   Delay in contraceptive effect – not effective until semen sample clear
   Failure – rejoining of vas deferens and fertility restoration: 0.2%–0.4% but can be up to 5%[8]
   Chronic testicular pain – up to 33% occasional testicular discomfort, 2% have significant pain[7]
   Granuloma due to leakage of sperm – 15%–40% but only 2%–3% are symptomatic[6]
   'Full' feeling due to filling of epididymis with stored sperm
   Procedure involves: Local anaesthesia (general anaesthesia is an option)

Key publications

Cook LA, Van Vliet H, Lopez LM, *et al.* Vasectomy occlusion techniques for male sterilisation. Cochrane Database Syst Rev. 2007; 2: CD003991.[9]

- Of the six studies meeting the inclusion criteria.
    - No difference in failure rates for clips vs. conventional vasectomy technique – one trial.
    - No difference in time to reach azoospermia between vasectomy and vas irrigation – three trials.
    - However the authors conclude that the above studies were of low quality and underpowered, thus the results cannot be accepted without further studies.
    - Comparison of fascial interposition vs. no fascial intervention showed a lower failure rate in the fascial interposition group. This group also had more surgical difficulties – one trial.
    - An intra-vas device had a lower success rate than no-scalpel vasectomy – 1 trial.

References

1 *No-scalpel Vasectomy: an illustrated guide for surgeons.* 2nd ed. New York: AVSC International; 1997.

2 Li SQ, Goldstein M, Zhu J, *et al.* The no-scalpel vasectomy. *J Urol.* 1991; **145**(2): 341–4.

3 Belker AM, Thomas AJ Jr, Fuchs EF, *et al.* Results of 1649 microsurgical vasectomy reversals by the Vasovasectomy Study Group. *J Urol.* 1991; **145**(3): 505–11.

4 Rosenberg MJ, Waugh MS. Latex condom breakage and slippage in a controlled clinical trial. *Contraception.* 1997; **56**: 17–21.

5 Kendrick JS, Gonzales B, Huber DH, *et al.* Complications of vasectomies in the United States. *J Fam Pract.* 1987; **25**(3): 245–8.

6 Peterson HB, Huber DH, Belker AM, *et al.* Vasectomy: an appraisal for the obstetrician-gynaecologist. *Obstet Gynecol.* 1990; **76**(3Pt2): 568–72.

7 Choe JM, Kirkemo AK. Questionnaire-based outcomes study of non-oncological post-vasectomy complications. *J Urol.* 1996; **155**(4): 1284–6.

8 Li SQ, Xu B, Hou YH, *et al.* Relationship between vas occlusion techniques and recanalization. *Adv Contracept Deliv Syst.* 1994; **10**: 153–9.

9 Cook LA, Van Vliet H, Lopez LM, *et al.* Vasectomy occlusion techniques for male sterilization. Cochrane Database Syst Rev. 2007; 2: CD003991.

Appendix A: Department of Health consent forms

The Department of Health have four published consent forms that are used in NHS hospitals throughout the UK. It is important to understand the purpose of each form in order use the most appropriate one.

Consent form 1 – Patient agreement to investigation or treatment

Consent form 2 – Parental agreement to investigation or treatment for a child or young person

Consent form 3 – Patient/parental agreement to investigation or treatment (where consciousness not impaired during the procedure)

Consent form 4 – Adults who are unable to consent to investigation or treatment

The following pages include sample consent forms 1, 2, 3 and 4 from the Department of Health (Reproduced under the terms of the Click-Use Licence).

Consent form 1: Patient agreement to investigation or treatment

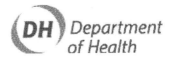

**[NHS organisation name]
consent form 1**

**Patient agreement to investigation
or treatment**

Patient details (or pre-printed label)

Patient's surname/family name.................................

Patient's first names ....

Date of birth ....

Responsible health professional..............................

Job title ....

NHS number (or other identifier)..............................

☐ Male   ☐ Female

Special requirements ....
(eg other language/other communication method)

To be retained in patient's notes

Patient identifier/label

Name of proposed procedure or course of treatment (include brief explanation if medical term not clear) ....
....
....

Statement of health professional (to be filled in by health professional with appropriate knowledge of proposed procedure, as specified in consent policy)

I have explained the procedure to the patient. In particular, I have explained:

The intended benefits ....
....
....
Serious or frequently occurring risks ....,,,,,   ,,,,.........................
.................................,,,,,   ,,,,,...
,,,,...
Any extra procedures which may become necessary during the procedure

☐ blood transfusion..

☐ other procedure (please specify) ....
....

I have also discussed what the procedure is likely to involve, the benefits and risks of any available alternative treatments (including no treatment) and any particular concerns of this patient.

☐ The following leaflet/tape has been provided ....

This procedure will involve:

☐ general and/or regional anaesthesia   ☐ local anaesthesia   ☐ sedation

Signed:..   Date .. ..
Name (PRINT) ....   Job title ....

Contact details (if patient wishes to discuss options later) ....

Statement of interpreter (where appropriate)

I have interpreted the information above to the patient to the best of my ability and in a way in which I believe s/he can understand.

Signed ....   Date ....
Name (PRINT) ....

Top copy accepted by patient: yes/no (please ring)

2

Statement of patient

Patient identifier/label

Please read this form carefully. If your treatment has been planned in advance, you should already have your own copy of page 2 which describes the benefits and risks of the proposed treatment. If not, you will be offered a copy now. If you have any further questions, do ask – we are here to help you. You have the right to change your mind at any time, including after you have signed this form.

I agree to the procedure or course of treatment described on this form.

I understand that you cannot give me a guarantee that a particular person will perform the procedure. The person will, however, have appropriate experience.

I understand that I will have the opportunity to discuss the details of anaesthesia with an anaesthetist before the procedure, unless the urgency of my situation prevents this. (This only applies to patients having general or regional anaesthesia.)

I understand that any procedure in addition to those described on this form will only be carried out if it is necessary to save my life or to prevent serious harm to my health.

I have been told about additional procedures which may become necessary during my treatment. I have listed below any procedures **which I do not wish to be carried out** without further discussion. ....
....
....
....

Patient's signature .... Date...............................
Name (PRINT) ....

A witness should sign below if the patient is unable to sign but has indicated his or her consent. Young people/children may also like a parent to sign here (see notes).

Signature .... Date ....
Name (PRINT) ....

Confirmation of consent (to be completed by a health professional when the patient is admitted for the procedure, if the patient has signed the form in advance)

On behalf of the team treating the patient, I have confirmed with the patient that s/he has no further questions and wishes the procedure to go ahead.

Signed:... Date ....
Name (PRINT) .... Job title ....

Important notes: (tick if applicable)

☐ See also advance directive/living will (eg Jehovah's Witness form)

☐ Patient has withdrawn consent (ask patient to sign /date here) ....

3

Guidance to health professionals (to be read in conjunction with consent policy)

What a consent form is for

This form documents the patient's agreement to go ahead with the investigation or treatment you have proposed. It is not a legal waiver – if patients, for example, do not receive enough information on which to base their decision, then the consent may not be valid, even though the form has been signed. Patients are also entitled to change their mind after signing the form, if they retain capacity to do so. The form should act as an *aide-memoire* to health professionals and patients, by providing a check-list of the kind of information patients should be offered, and by enabling the patient to have a written record of the main points discussed. In no way, however, should the written information provided for the patient be regarded as a substitute for face-to-face discussions with the patient.

The law on consent

See the Department of Health's *Reference guide to consent for examination or treatment* for a comprehensive summary of the law on consent (also available at www.doh.gov.uk/consent).

Who can give consent

Everyone aged 16 or more is presumed to be competent to give consent for themselves, unless the opposite is demonstrated. If a child under the age of 16 has "sufficient understanding and intelligence to enable him or her to understand fully what is proposed", then he or she will be competent to give consent for himself or herself. Young people aged 16 and 17, and legally 'competent' younger children, may therefore sign this form for themselves, but may like a parent to countersign as well. If the child is not able to give consent for himself or herself, some-one with parental responsibility may do so on their behalf and a separate form is available for this purpose. Even where a child is able to give consent for himself or herself, you should always involve those with parental responsibility in the child's care, unless the child specifically asks you not to do so. If a patient is mentally competent to give consent but is physically unable to sign a form, you should complete this form as usual, and ask an independent witness to confirm that the patient has given consent orally or non-verbally.

When NOT to use this form

If the patient is 18 or over and is not legally competent to give consent, you should use form 4 (form for adults who are unable to consent to investigation or treatment) instead of this form. A patient will not be legally competent to give consent if:
• they are unable to comprehend and retain information material to the decision and/or
• they are unable to weigh and use this information in coming to a decision.
You should always take all reasonable steps (for example involving more specialist colleagues) to support a patient in making their own decision, before concluding that they are unable to do so. Relatives **cannot** be asked to sign this form on behalf of an adult who is not legally competent to consent for himself or herself.

Information

Information about what the treatment will involve, its benefits and risks (including side-effects and complications) and the alternatives to the particular procedure proposed, is crucial for patients when making up their minds. The courts have stated that patients should be told about 'significant risks which would affect the judgement of a reasonable patient'. 'Significant' has not been legally defined, but the GMC requires doctors to tell patients about 'serious or frequently occurring' risks. In addition if patients make clear they have particular concerns about certain kinds of risk, you should make sure they are informed about these risks, even if they are very small or rare. You should always answer questions honestly. Sometimes, patients may make it clear that they do not want to have any information about the options, but want you to decide on their behalf. In such circumstances, you should do your best to ensure that the patient receives at least very basic information about what is proposed. Where information is refused, you should document this on page 2 of the form or in the patient's notes.

4

146

Consent form 2: Parental agreement to investigation or treatment for a child or young person

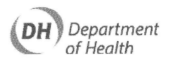

[NHS organisation name]
consent form 2

Parental agreement to investigation or treatment for a child or young person

---

Patient details (or pre-printed label)

Patient's surname/family name.................................

Patient's first names ....

Date of birth ....

Age ....

Responsible health professional................................

Job title ....

NHS number (or other identifier)................................

☐ Male   ☐ Female

Special requirements ....
(eg other language/other communication method)

To be retained in patient's notes

Patient identifier/label

Name of proposed procedure or course of treatment (include brief

explanation if medical term not clear) ....

....

....

Statement of health professional (to be filled in by health professional with

appropriate knowledge of proposed procedure, as specified in consent policy)

I have explained the procedure to the child and his or her parent(s). In particular, I have explained:

The intended benefits ....

....

Serious or frequently occurring risks ....

....

....

Any extra procedures which may become necessary during the procedure

☐ blood transfusion...

☐ other procedure (please specify) ....

....

I have also discussed what the procedure is likely to involve, the benefits and risks of any available alternative treatments (including no treatment) and any particular concerns of this patient and his or her parents.

☐ The following leaflet/tape has been provided ....

This procedure will involve:

☐ general and/or regional anaesthesia   ☐ local anaesthesia   ☐ sedation

Signed:..   Date ....
Name (PRINT) ....   Job title ....

Contact details (if child/parent wish to discuss options later) ....

Statement of interpreter (where appropriate)

I have interpreted the information above to the child and his or her parents to the best of my ability and in a way in which I believe they can understand.

Signed ....   Date ....
Name (PRINT) ....

Top copy accepted by patient: yes/no (please ring)

2

Statement of parent

Patient identifier/label

Please read this form carefully. If the procedure has been planned in advance, you should already have your own copy of page 2 which describes the benefits and risks of the proposed treatment. If not, you will be offered a copy now. If you have any further questions, do ask – we are here to help you and your child. You have the right to change your mind at any time, including after you have signed this form.

I agree to the procedure or course of treatment described on this form and **I confirm** that I have 'parental responsibility' for this child.

I understand that you cannot give me a guarantee that a particular person will perform the procedure. The person will, however, have appropriate experience.

I understand that my child and I will have the opportunity to discuss the details of anaesthesia with an anaesthetist before the procedure, unless the urgency of the situation prevents this. (This only applies to children having general or regional anaesthesia.)

I understand hat any procedure in addition to those described on this form will only be carried out if it is necessary to save the life of my child or to prevent serious harm to his or her health.

I have been told about additional procedures which may become necessary during my child's treatment. I have listed below any **procedures which I do not wish to be carried out** without further discussion. ....
....
....
....

Signature .... Date...............................
Name (PRINT) ....Relationship to child................................

Child's agreement to treatment (if child wishes to sign)

I agree to have the treatment I have been told about.

Name .... Signature ....
Date ....

Confirmation of consent (to be completed by a health professional when the child is admitted for the procedure, if the parent/child have signed the form in advance)

On behalf of the team treating the patient, I have confirmed with the child and his or her parent(s) that they have no further questions and wish the procedure to go ahead.

Signed:.. Date ....
Name (PRINT) .... Job title ....

Important notes: (tick if applicable)

☐ See also advance directive/living will (eg Jehovah's Witness form)

☐ Parent has withdrawn consent (ask parent to sign /date here) ....

3

Guidance to health professionals (to be read in conjunction with consent policy)

This form

This form should be used to document consent to a child's treatment, where that consent is being given by a person with parental responsibility for the child. The term 'parent' has been used in this form as a shorthand for 'person with parental responsibility'. Where children are legally competent to consent for themselves (see below), they may sign the standard 'adult' consent form (form 1). There is space on that form for a parent to countersign if a competent child wishes them to do so.

Who can give consent

Everyone aged 16 or more is presumed to be competent to give consent for themselves, unless the opposite is demonstrated. The courts have stated that if a child under the age of 16 has "sufficient understanding and intelligence to enable him or her to understand fully what is proposed", then he or she will be competent to give consent for himself or herself. If children are not able to give consent for themselves, some-one with parental responsibility may do so on their behalf.

Although children acquire rights to give consent for themselves as they grow older, people with 'parental responsibility' for a child retain the right to give consent on the child's behalf until the child reaches the age of 18. Therefore, for a number of years, both the child and a person with parental responsibility have the right to give consent to the child's treatment. In law, health professionals only need the consent of one appropriate person before providing treatment. This means that in theory it is lawful to provide treatment to a child under 18 which a person with parental responsibility has authorised, even if the child refuses. As a matter of good practice, however, you should always seek a competent child's consent before providing treatment unless any delay involved in doing so would put the child's life or health at risk. Younger children should also be as involved as possible in decisions about their healthcare. Further advice is given in the Department's guidance *Seeking consent: working with children*. Any differences of opinion between the child and their parents, or between parents, should be clearly documented in the patient's notes.

Parental responsibility

The person(s) with parental responsibility will usually, but not invariably, be the child's birth parents. People with parental responsibility for a child include: the child's mother; the child's father if married to the mother at the child's conception, birth or later; a legally appointed guardian; the local authority if the child is on a care order; or a person named in a residence order in respect of the child. Fathers who have never been married to the child's mother will only have parental responsibility if they have acquired it through a court order or parental responsibility agreement (although this may change in the future).

Information

Information about what the treatment will involve, its benefits and risks (including side-effects and complications) and the alternatives to the particular procedure proposed, is crucial for children and their parents when making up their minds about treatment. The courts have stated that patients should be told about 'significant risks which would affect the judgement of a reasonable patient'. 'Significant' has not been legally defined, but the GMC requires doctors to tell patients about 'serious or frequently occurring' risks. In addition if patients make clear they have particular concerns about certain kinds of risk, you should make sure they are informed about these risks, even if they are very small or rare. You should always answer questions honestly.

Guidance on the law on consent

See the Department of Health publications *Reference guide to consent for examination or treatment* and *Seeking consent: working with children* for a comprehensive summary of the law on consent (also available at www.doh.gov.uk/consent).

4

Consent form 3: Patient/parental agreement to investigation or treatment

[NHS organisation name] consent form 3

Patient identifier/label

Patient/parental agreement to investigation or treatment
(procedures where consciousness not impaired)

Name of procedure (include brief explanation if medical term not clear)
....
....

Statement of health professional (to be filled in by health professional with appropriate knowledge of proposed procedure, as specified in consent policy)

I have explained the procedure to the patient/parent. In particular, I have explained:
The intended benefits ....
....
....
Serious or frequently occurring risks:..
....
....

I have also discussed what the procedure is likely to involve, the benefits and risks of any available alternative treatments (including no treatment) and any particular concerns of those involved.

☐ The following leaflet/tape has been provided ....

Signed: .... Date ....
Name (PRINT) .... Job title ....

Statement of interpreter (where appropriate)
I have interpreted the information above to the patient/parent to the best of my ability and in a way in which I believe s/he/they can understand.

Signed ....Date....................Name (PRINT)...................................

Statement of patient/person with parental responsibility for patient
I agree to the procedure described above.

I understand that you cannot give me a guarantee that a particular person will perform the procedure. The person will, however, have appropriate experience.

I understand that the procedure will/will not involve local anaesthesia.

Signature .... Date ....
Name (PRINT) .... Relationship to patient ....

Confirmation of consent (to be completed by a health professional when the patient is admitted for the procedure, if the patient/parent has signed the form in advance)

I have confirmed that the patient/parent has no further questions and wishes the procedure to go ahead.

Signed: .... Date ....
Name (PRINT) .... Job title ....

Top copy accepted by patient: yes/no (please ring)

Guidance to health professionals (to be read in conjunction with consent policy)

This form
This form documents the patient's agreement (or that of a person with parental responsibility for the patient) to go ahead with the investigation or treatment you have proposed. **It is only designed for procedures where the patient is expected to remain alert throughout and where an anaesthetist is not involved in their care: for example for drug therapy where written consent is deemed appropriate.** In other circumstances you should use either form 1 (for adults/competent children) or form 2 (parental consent for children/young people) as appropriate.

Consent forms are not legal waivers – if patients, for example, do not receive enough information on which to base their decision, then the consent may not be valid, even though the form has been signed. Patients also have every right to change their mind after signing the form.

Who can give consent
Everyone aged 16 or more is presumed to be competent to give consent for themselves, unless the opposite is demonstrated. If a child under the age of 16 has "sufficient understanding and intelligence to enable him or her to understand fully what is proposed", then he or she will be competent to give consent for himself or herself. Young people aged 16 and 17, and legally 'competent' younger children, may therefore sign this form for themselves, if they wish. If the child is not able to give consent for himself or herself, some-one with parental responsibility may do so on their behalf. Even where a child is able to give consent for himself or herself, you should always involve those with parental responsibility in the child's care, unless the child specifically asks you not to do so. If a patient is mentally competent to give consent but is physically unable to sign a form, you should complete this form as usual, and ask an independent witness to confirm that the patient has given consent orally or non-verbally.

When NOT to use this form (see also 'This form' above)
If the patient is 18 or over and is not legally competent to give consent, you should use form 4 (form for adults who are unable to consent to investigation or treatment) instead of this form. A patient will not be legally competent to give consent if:
• they are unable to comprehend and retain information material to the decision and/or
• they are unable to weigh and use this information in coming to a decision.
You should always take all reasonable steps (for example involving more specialist colleagues) to support a patient in making their own decision, before concluding that they are unable to do so. Relatives **cannot** be asked to sign this form on behalf of an adult who is not legally competent to consent for himself or herself.

Information
Information about what the treatment will involve, its benefits and risks (including side-effects and complications) and the alternatives to the particular procedure proposed, is crucial for patients when making up their minds about treatment. The courts have stated that patients should be told about 'significant risks which would affect the judgement of a reasonable patient'. 'Significant' has not been legally defined, but the GMC requires doctors to tell patients about 'serious or frequently occurring' risks. In addition if patients make clear they have particular concerns about certain kinds of risk, you should make sure they are informed about these risks, even if they are very small or rare. You should always answer questions honestly. Sometimes, patients may make it clear that they do not want to have any information about the options, but want you to decide on their behalf. In such circumstances, you should do your best to ensure that the patient receives at least very basic information about what is proposed. Where information is refused, you should document this overleaf or in the patient's notes.

The law on consent
See the Department of Health's *Reference guide to consent for examination or treatment* for a comprehensive summary of the law on consent (also available at www.doh.gov.uk/consent).

Consent form 4: Adults who are unable to consent to investigation or treatmenta

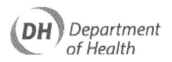

[NHS organisation name]
consent form 4

Form for adults who are unable to consent to investigation or treatment

---

Patient details (or pre-printed label)

Patient's surname/family name................................

Patient's first names ....

Date of birth ....

Responsible health professional................................

Job title ....

NHS number (or other identifier).................................

☐ Male   ☐ Female

Special requirements ....
(eg other language/other communication method)

To be retained in patient's notes

Patient identifier/label

All sections to be completed by health professional proposing the procedure

A Details of procedure or course of treatment proposed

(NB see guidance to health professionals overleaf for details of situations where court approval must first be sought)

B Assessment of patient's capacity

I confirm that the patient lacks capacity to give or withhold consent to this procedure or course of treatment because:

the patient is unable to comprehend and retain information material to the decision; and/or

the patient is unable to use and weigh this information in the decision-making process; or

the patient is unconscious

Further details (excluding where patient unconscious): for example how above judgements reached; which colleagues consulted; what attempts made to assist the patient make his or her own decision and why these were not successful.

C Assessment of patient's best interests

To the best of my knowledge, the patient has not refused this procedure in a valid advance directive. Where possible and appropriate, I have consulted with colleagues and those close to the patient, and I believe the procedure to be in the patient's best interests because:

(Where incapacity is likely to be temporary, for example if patient unconscious, or where patient has fluctuating capacity)

The treatment cannot wait until the patient recovers capacity because:

2

D Involvement of the patient's family and others close to the patient

The final responsibility for determining whether a procedure is in an incapacitated patient's best interests lies with the health professional performing the procedure. However, it is good practice to consult with those close to the patient (eg spouse/partner, family and friends, carer, supporter or advocate) unless you have good reason to believe that the patient would not have wished particular individuals to be consulted, or unless the urgency of their situation prevents this. "Best interests" go far wider than "best medical interests", and include factors such as the patient's wishes and beliefs when competent, their current wishes, their general well-being and their spiritual and religious welfare.

(to be signed by a person or persons close to the patient, if they wish)

I/We have been involved in a discussion with the relevant health professionals over the treatment of..............................(patient's name). I/We understand that he/she is unable to give his/her own consent, based on the criteria set out in this form. I/We also understand that treatment can lawfully be provided if it is in his/her best interests to receive it.

Any other comments (including any concerns about decision)

Name ....Relationship to patient.....................................
Address (if not the same as patient...
....
....

Signature .... Date.............................

If a person close to the patient was not available in person, has this matter been discussed in any other way (eg over the telephone?)

☐ Yes   ☐ No
Details:

Signature of health professional proposing treatment

The above procedure is, in my clinical judgement, in the best interests of the patient, who lacks capacity to consent for himself or herself. Where possible and appropriate I have discussed the patient's condition with those close to him or her, and taken their knowledge of the patient's views and beliefs into account in determining his or her best interests.

I have/have not sought a second opinion.

Signature:.. Date .. ..
Name (PRINT) .... Job title ....

Where second opinion sought, s/he should sign below to confirm agreement:

Signature:.. Date .. ..
Name (PRINT) .... Job title ....

3

155

Guidance to health professionals (to be read in conjunction with consent policy)

This form should only be used where it would be usual to seek written consent but an adult patient (18 or over) lacks capacity to give or withhold consent to treatment. If an adult **has** capacity to accept or refuse treatment, you should use the standard consent form and respect any refusal. Where treatment is very urgent (for example if the patient is critically ill), it may not be feasible to fill in a form at the time, but you should document your clinical decisions appropriately afterwards. If treatment is being provided under the authority of Part IV of the *Mental Health Act 1983*, different legal provisions apply and you are required to fill in more specialised forms (although in some circumstances you may find it helpful to use this form as well). If the adult now lacks capacity, but has clearly refused particular treatment in advance of their loss of capacity (for example in an advance directive or 'living will'), then you must abide by that refusal if it was validly made and is applicable to the circumstances. For further information on the law on consent, see the Department of Health's *Reference guide to consent for examination or treatment* (www.doh.gov.uk/consent).

When treatment can be given to a patient who is unable to consent
For treatment to be given to a patient who is unable to consent, the following **must** apply:
•• the patient must lack the capacity ('competence') to give or withhold consent to this procedure AND
•• the procedure must be in the patient's best interests.

Capacity
A patient will lack capacity to consent to a particular intervention if he or she is:
•• unable to comprehend and retain information material to the decision, especially as to the consequences of having, or not having, the intervention in question; and/or
•• unable to use and weigh this information in the decision-making process.
Before making a judgement that a patient lacks capacity you must take all steps reasonable in the circumstances to assist the patient in taking their own decisions (this will clearly not apply if the patient is unconscious). This may involve explaining what is involved in very simple language, using pictures and communication and decision-aids as appropriate. People close to the patient (spouse/partner, family, friends and carers) may often be able to help, as may specialist colleagues such as speech and language therapists or learning disability teams, and independent advocates or supporters.

Capacity is 'decision-specific': a patient may lack capacity to take a particular complex decision, but be quite able to take other more straight-forward decisions or parts of decisions.

Best interests
A patient's best interests are not limited to their best medical interests. Other factors which form part of the best interests decision include:
•• the wishes and beliefs of the patient when competent
•• their current wishes
•• their general well-being
•• their spiritual and religious welfare

Two incapacitated patients, whose *physical* condition is identical, may therefore have different best interests.

Unless the patient has clearly indicated that particular individuals should not be involved in their care, or unless the urgency of their situation prevents it, you should attempt to involve people close to the patient (spouse/partner, family and friends, carer, supporter or advocate) in the decision-making process. Those close to the patient cannot require you to provide particular treatment which you do not believe to be clinically appropriate. However they will know the patient much better than you do, and therefore are likely to be able to provide valuable information about the patient's wishes and values.

Second opinions and court involvement
Where treatment is complex and/or people close to the patient express doubts about the proposed treatment, a second opinion should be sought, unless the urgency of the patient's condition prevents this. Donation of regenerative tissue such as bone marrow, sterilisation for contraceptive purposes and withdrawal of artificial nutrition or hydration from a patient in PVS must never be undertaken without prior High Court approval. High Court approval can also be sought where there are doubts about the patient's capacity or best interests.

4

Appendix B: Laparoscopy and laparotomy

Laparoscopy
Key Points
Laparoscopy is the examination of the abdominal cavity with a laparoscope. It has been performed for over a century, although widespread credence occurred only when the technology was synthesised with video to permit projection of the intraoperative image. In a relatively short time, laparoscopic techniques have been adapted to a wide range of general surgical scenarios from cholecystectomy and hernia repair to major colonic cancer resection. In the era of minimally invasive surgery, the advantages to patients and practitioners are clear: smaller more cosmetically acceptable incisions; less pain; quicker recovery time and reduced length of hospital stay.

The diagnostic laparoscopy
Interventional laparoscopy is increasingly common, however in certain circumstances it is also a useful diagnostic tool. The procedure permits inspection of intra-abdominal organs as well as the acquisition of histological and microbiological specimens and can also be used in conjunction with ultrasound to examine structures that cannot be visualised directly.

Diagnostic laparoscopy is well established in the staging of certain cancers (particularly in hepatobiliary surgery). For the surgeon-in-training, however, it may be more frequently performed in the context of unexplained acute abdominal pain. The Society of American Gastrointestinal and Laparoscopic Surgeons (SAGES) guidelines suggest that diagnostic laparoscopy may be superior to close observation for patients with non-specific abdominal pain whose diagnosis remains unclear after all non-invasive diagnostic channels have been exhausted. However, it is acknowledged that on this point, the evidence is conflicting. The literature suggests that although the time to diagnosis and hospital stay may be shortened, the morbidity associated with diagnostic laparoscopy may be as high as 24% (including trocar injury, wound infection, ileus and pelvic collections amongst others).[1]

Laparoscopic entry techniques
Many of the major complications associated with laparoscopy are related to port entry. The incidence of trocar injury to major blood vessels and to bowel is 0.9/1000 and 1.8/1000 respectively.[2]

There are a number of methods of port entry in use. Traditionally, gynaecologists have preferred to use the Veress needle; an insufflation device with a spring-loaded obturator which encloses the tip once the peritoneum has been breached. In contrast general surgeons are more comfortable with open approaches, whereby the peritoneum is penetrated with sharp dissection, under direct vision.

As trocar-related complications are rare, most of the studies comparing different entry techniques are underpowered and it is perhaps unsurprising that a meta-analysis of 17 RCTs failed establish a superior method.[2]

The future?

The rapid development of laparoscopic surgery has been mirrored by similar advances in flexible endoscopy. The amalgamation of these technologies may herald the next step in the evolution of minimally invasive surgery, leading to even less invasive operations. NOTES (Natural Orifice Transluminal Endoscopic Surgery) is performed by instrumentation through the body's pre-existing orifices. At this stage, numerous operations have been trialled in animal models but this has yet to translate into widespread use in humans.[3]

References

1 Society of American Gastrointestinal and Endoscopic Surgeons. Diagnostic laparoscopy guidelines. *Surg Endosc.* 2008; **22***:* 1353–83.
2 Ahmad G, Duffy JMN, Phillips K, *et al.* Laparoscopic entry techniques. Cochrane Database Syst Rev. 2008; 2: CD006583.
3 Rattner D, Kalloo A. ASGE/SAGES working group on natural orifice transluminal endoscopic surgery. *Surg Endosc.* 2006; **20***:* 329–33.

Laparotomy
Key Points

Laparotomy is an incision through the abdominal wall used in vascular, urological, gynaecological and general surgery. It was the only means of access to the abdominal and retroperitoneal viscera, prior to the introduction of laparoscopic and endoluminal techniques.

In the emergency setting, the term laparotomy usually signifies an exploratory midline incision, to diagnose and treat pathology in the context of blunt or penetrating trauma, generalised peritonitis, intestinal obstruction, aneurysm rupture or gastrointestinal bleeding.

Laparotomy incisions

* Midline: quick, minimises bleeding, easy to extend, and provides good general access to the abdomen, pelvis and retroperitoneal structures.
* Paramedian: a vertical incision offset from the midline, achieved by drawing the rectus sheath laterally. Also provides good general access to the abdomen.
* Oblique: these are targeted incisions. The gridiron and Rutherford Morison incisions are useful for right-sided colonic pathology. Kocher's subcostal approach is used in hepatic and biliary surgery and can be extended across the midline in a rooftop configuration.
* Transverse: transverse scars usually have a better cosmetic appearance. The Lanz approach is popular for appendicitis and the Pfannenstiel incision for access to pelvic organs. Midabdominal transverse incisions are sometime preferred by vascular surgeons to access the major abdominal vessels.

The midline laparotomy

The skin incision is centred in the upper or lower midline depending on the site of the pathology. It can be extended cranially or caudally by circumventing the umbilicus.

The subcutaneous fat is divided to expose the linea alba. The aponeurosis is divided with a knife, exposing preperitoneal fat. The peritoneum is drawn up between two artery forceps, (taking care not to catch the viscera beneath), before it too is divided with the belly of a knife. Once the peritoneum has been breached, the abdominal contents fall away, permitting careful extension of the wound as required.

Wound-related complications include infection, dehiscence and hernia formation. In order to minimise these, mass closure is the technique of choice; incorporating all of the layers of the abdominal wall (except skin) as a single structure, in a simple running technique, using #1 or #2 absorbable monofilament suture material with a suture-length to wound-length ratio of 4 to 1.[1]

Reference

1 Ceydeli A, Rucinski J, Wise L. Finding the best abdominal closure: an evidence-based review of the literature. *Curr Surg*. 2005; **62**: 220–5.

Index